GLUTEN FREE COOKBOOK

The Ultimate Gluten Free Diet Cookbook for Busy People - Gluten Free Recipes for Weight Loss, Energy, and Optimum Health

© Copyright 2017 - All rights reserved.

The contents of this book may not be reproduced, duplicated or transmitted without direct written permission from the author.

Under no circumstances will any legal responsibility or blame be held against the publisher for any reparation, damages, or monetary loss due to the information herein, either directly or indirectly.

Legal Notice:

This book is copyright protected. This is only for personal use. You cannot amend, distribute, sell, use, quote or paraphrase any part or the content within this book without the consent of the author.

Disclaimer Notice:

Please note the information contained within this document is for educational and entertainment purposes only. Every attempt has been made to provide accurate, up to date and reliable complete information. No warranties of any kind are expressed or implied. Readers acknowledge that the author is not engaging in the rendering of legal, financial, medical or professional advice. The content of this book has been derived from various sources. Please consult a licensed professional before attempting any techniques outlined in this book.

By reading this document, the reader agrees that under no circumstances are is the author responsible for any losses, direct or indirect, which are incurred as a result of the use of information contained within this document, including, but not limited to, —errors, omissions, or inaccuracies.

Table of Contents

Introduction 6
Chapter 1: What is the Gluten Free Diet? 7
Chapter 2: The Health Benefits of the Gluten Free Diet 12
Chapter 3: Case Studies of Gluten Free Diets Working 15
Chapter 4: Foods to Eat and Foods to Avoid 19
Chapter 5: Gluten Free Appetizers & Snacks Recipes 22
    Refreshing Fresh Tomato Salsa 22
    BLT Style Dip 23
    Delicious Ham and Cream Cheese Roll Ups with Dill Pickle 24
    Quick and Easy Guacamole 25
    Buffalo Chicken Wings 26
    Creamy and Tangy Cilantro Sauce 27
    Traditional Hummus 28
    Gluten Free Artichoke and Spinach Dip 29
    Buttery and Tangy Grilled Basil Shrimp 30
    Grilled Marinated Shrimp 31
    Healthy Baked Kale Chips 32
    Spiced Pumpkin Seeds 33
Chapter 6: Breakfast and Brunch Recipes 34
    Eggs with Zucchini 34
    Delicious and Healthy Gluten Free Pancakes 35
    Gluten Free Ham and Cheese Breakfast Quiche 36
    Quick Greek Style Scrambled Eggs 37
    Baby Spinach Omelet 38
    Sautéed Cinnamon Apples 39
    Country Style Fried Potatoes 40
    Healthy Corned Beef Hash 41
    Oven Roasted Rosemary Butter New Potato Wedges 42
    Scrambled Feta Eggs 43
Chapter 7: Meal Recipes 44
    Gluten Free Shrimp Creole 44
    Baked Egg and Veggie Pie 46

Grilled Teriyaki Flank Steak 47
Easy Grilled Chicken Breast with Grilled Vegetables and Bacon 48
Buttery Grilled Sea Bass 49
Gluten Free Whole Roasted Chicken 50
Gluten Free Cheese and Herb Pizza Crust 51
Quinoa Stuffed Pork Tenderloin 53
Caramel Apple Pork Chops 55
Slow Cooked Pulled BBQ Pork 56
Cabbage Roll Casserole 57
Infallible Rib Roast 58
Beef and Rice Stuffed Peppers 59
Blackened Chicken 60
Lamb Chops with Balsamic Reduction 61
Slow Cooked Hot Mexican Style Meat 62
Spicy and Tangy Chicken Kabobs 63
Cornish Game Hens with Garlic and Rosemary 64
Delicious Dill Chickpea Sandwich Filling 66
Garlic Butter Sirloin Steak 67
Slow Cooked Barbeque Chuck Roast 68

Chapter 8: Bread & Side Recipes 69

Fluffy Gluten Free Cornbread 69
Gluten Free Banana Bread 70
Gluten Free Zucchini Bread 71
Gluten Free Bread Machine White Bread 73
Gluten Free Irish Soda Bread 74
Pao de Queijo – The Brazilian Cheese Bread 75
Light and Fluffy Cloud Bread 76
Roasted Brussels sprouts 77
Grilled Asparagus Spears 78
Green Beans with Cherry Tomatoes 79
Spicy Quinoa with Corn and Black Beans 80
Tangy Harvest Rice Dish 81
Buttery Green Beans with Garlic 82
Boston Baked Beans 83
Slow Cooked Creamed Corn 84
Oven Roasted Sugar Snap Peas 85
Creamy Roasted Garlic Mashed Potatoes 86
Pan Tossed White Wine and Italian Herbed Mushrooms 87

Chapter 9: Dessert Recipes 88

Chocolate Dipped Coconut Bon-Bons 88
Delicious Gluten Free Layer Bars 89
Delicious Chocolate and Cream Cheese Fudge 90
Delicious Gluten Free Orange Cake 91
Gluten Free Coconut Macaroons 93
Gluten Free Flourless Chocolate Cake 94
Delicious Chocolate Meringue Cookies 95
Zingy Lemon Soufflé 96
Gluten Free Peanut Butter Cookies 98
Gooey Black Bean Brownies 99
Gluten Free Garbanzo Bean Chocolate Cake 100
Creamy Gluten Free Rice Pudding 101
Cream Cheese Mints 102

Chapter 10: Common Units of Conversion in the Kitchen 103
US Dry Volume Measurements 103
US liquid volume measurements 103
US to Metric Conversions 104
Metric to US Conversions 104
Oven Temperature Conversions 104

Conclusion 105

Introduction

Unless you've been living under a rock for the past few years, you must have heard about the gluten-free diet. However, despite its quick rise to popularity, not many people are clear what the diet entails.

Gluten is a protein present in grains; many people aren't able to digest it. It is also a major component in most processed foods. The gluten-free diet calls for the avoidance of those foods and promotes the consumption of healthy, natural and unprocessed foods.

The gluten-free diet has been the source of a lot of speculation and debates through the time since it was introduced. Some physicians, nutritionists and dieticians stand by the diet, while others claim that it's a sham. Well, I assure you it is not a sham! There are loads of people who have followed this diet and have had their lives change for good - from losing weight to getting clear skin, improved digestion, better sleep, reduction of anxiety, etc. When you go gluten-free, you cut out a lot of unhealthy foods, fried foods and processed foods from your diet. These foods are usually cited to be detrimental to your health, so how does a diet that makes you avoid these foods be bad or unhealthy?

In this book, you will find a lot of details about the diet, from an in-depth explanation of what the diet entails, its benefits, success stories of people who followed the diet and achieved great results, the foods you should eat and the ones you should avoid and a whole bunch of recipes that will help you become a gluten free Master Chef in your kitchen. All this with minimum efforts and using simple ingredients that are commonly available in most households. At the end of this book, there is also a conversion chart for common kitchen measurements and other conversions you may need in the kitchen.

If you do not believe in the gluten free diet or believe it's a sham, I assure you that, by the time you reach the end of this book, you will be a believer! I would like to take this opportunity to thank you for purchasing this book and I hope you find the contents of this book helpful.

Happy cooking!

Chapter 1: What is the Gluten Free Diet?

The Gluten free diet is pretty self-explanatory – it is a diet that calls for the avoidance of the consumption of gluten. Gluten is a protein that is normally found in most grains like wheat, rye, barley and triticale - the hybrid grain that is a result of a cross between rye and wheat.

The gluten free diet is essentially used to cure celiac disease. People who suffer from celiac disease have an inflammation of the small intestine every time gluten enters their digestive track. When gluten is eliminated from their diet, all the symptoms of celiac disease reduce drastically and this results in the prevention of further complications to their health.

A lot of people don't suffer from celiac disease but experience certain symptoms usually associated with celiac disease when they consume gluten. This kind of gluten intolerance is known as the non-celiac gluten sensitivity.

People who suffer from non-celiac gluten sensitivity don't necessarily need to follow the gluten-free diet but, if they do, they will find that their symptoms are abated and they feel relief. But people who do suffer from celiac disease absolutely need to cut gluten from their diet in order to inhibit the symptoms associated with the disease and prevent any further complications that can be serious if left unchecked.

Initially, you may find it a little difficult and even frustrating to follow the gluten-free diet. It is a big change and it will take some time for your mind and body to adjust to this change. The dietary restrictions may seem extremely stringent and rather pointless to people who do not suffer from extreme symptoms.

But, with a little patience and time you will easily adjust to the diet – rather, you will even find that most of the foods that you usually consume are gluten free and you will also be able to find delicious and gluten free substitutes for the gluten-filled foods that you like. With the demand for gluten-free products on a rise, there are various gluten free substitutes for traditional bread and pasta available on the market. It also helps in adjusting to the new diet, when you focus on the foods that you can consume, rather than focusing on the foods you cannot consume.

When you begin the gluten-free diet, it is important that you consult a trained dietician.

They can help you with a lot of things – like preparing a well-balanced diet plan, give you advice and answer all your queries pertaining to the diet.

Top 5 mistakes people make while going gluten free

Maybe because celiac diagnosis is at an all-time high, or because more and more people are choosing to eat healthy food and follow a healthy lifestyle, the number of people following the gluten-free diet is on a rise.

The gluten-free diet can have a huge impact on your health and provide you with a number of benefits, but only if you do it right!

If you do not remove gluten completely from your diet, you won't be able to reap all the benefits of the diet. Rather, you will find little to no change in your body! Here is a list of top 5 mistakes that people make when they embark on the gluten free diet and how you can avoid them for a glitch-free experience:

1. *Not having adequate information regarding the foods that contain gluten*

This is one of the most common mistakes people make when they go gluten free. You already know that gluten is a protein that is present in grains like wheat, barley, rye, etc. but these ingredients are often marketed under other names, making it difficult to keep track of them. When people think of gluten free, they think, "I have to avoid bread and pasta etc." but did you know that products like licorice and soy sauce also contain gluten?

This is why it is important to read labels and know what to look for. Chapter 4 talks in detail about the foods you need to avoid and the various ingredients that you need to look out for on labels!

2. *Consuming large amounts of gluten free foods that are highly processed*

Due to the rise in the popularity of the gluten-free diet, there has also been a rise in the demand for gluten-free products on the market. Since this is a strict diet, people usually find it difficult to transition from a regular diet to a gluten free diet. Cue in gluten-free processed foods that help you with the transition. But, what people don't really realize is that these foods are even less nutritious than their gluten-containing counterparts and can wreak havoc on the body due to their high fat and sugar content.

Also, the foods that are marketed as "gluten free" can by law contain about 20 parts per million or less. This quantity is too small to bother you if ingested on occasion, but if you consume a large amount of those foods, there is a gradual buildup of gluten in the body, undoing all your progress. So, stay as away from "gluten free" labeled foods as you can.

3. *Not consuming enough of the high-quality gluten free foods*

Many people switch to a gluten free diet plan to battle health issues – from celiac disease to autism, to Crohn's disease, to skin problems. Instead of simply doing away with gluten-containing processed foods and opting for gluten-containing processed foods, opt for natural foods like dairy, fruits, vegetables, eggs, meat, nuts, fish, seeds, etc.

These natural foods reduce the inflammation in the body and can make you feel good from the inside. They will also help you lose weight and provide your body with much-needed nutrients.

4. *Not taking supplements or cosmetics into consideration*

This is a mistake made by most people who usually don't deal with food restrictions. This results in the accidental consumption of gluten, without them even knowing it!

Yes, you do not eat your cosmetics, but the products still do enter your body – especially lip and eye products. These products usually have vitamin E that is extracted from wheat germ!

Quite a lot of the time, vitamins and supplements have gluten in them to retain their elasticity. So, read the labels and look for substitutes when required!

5. *Not being aware of cross-contamination*

Before shifting to the gluten free diet not many people realize that how little of an allergen is needed to cause a reaction. Cross contamination can be dangerous for people who suffer from celiac disease or gluten intolerance, as it takes as little 50 ppm of gluten to trigger a reaction in the body.

The next section explains cross contamination in great detail and the steps that you can take to avoid it from happening.

Mistakes are a part and parcel of life, but if you are forewarned, you know what precautions you can take to prevent them! Now, that you know what the common mistakes are, you can easily avoid them and make your gluten free experience hitch free!

Cross Contamination

Cross-contamination is when a gluten-free food comes into contact with food that contains gluten. There are various ways in which cross contamination may happen:

Cross contamination during manufacturing

Cross contamination is possible at the manufacturing level. There are three common ways in which cross contamination happens at the manufacturing level:

1. **Dusting** – Manufacturers of sticky foods, such as dried fruits, dust the foods with small quantities of wheat or oat flour to prevent sticking. This is usually listed in the "contains" or "allergens" section, check the labels before buying as seemingly gluten-free foods could contain gluten!

2. **Equipment** – Often a single manufacturing unit may manufacture multiple food items using the same equipment and machinery. The equipment and machinery may not necessarily be cleaned between producing two products. This may lead to cross contamination.

3. **Single Plant, Multiple Products** – A plant may have separate dedicated equipment and areas to keep allergens away from other foods, but this may not necessarily prevent airborne ingredients from flying around. For example, wheat flour may become airborne during a dough mixing process and may come into contact with gluten free foods.

Even though there is a law that states that all food products need to carry a gluten warning on them, there are certain loopholes that aid the manufacturer to work around the law; such as the "may contain" warning which is voluntary.

Also, according to the FDA guidelines, any food that has less than 20 ppm (parts per million) of gluten can carry the gluten free label. But, products labeled "wheat free" have no such guideline.

In this case, it is extremely important that you closely read the labels of everything you buy, and if you are not sure about the product's gluten content – buy a substitute or contact the manufacturer for details!

Cross contamination at home

It is not necessary that just because you have decided to go gluten free the rest of your family, your partner or your roommate will join you in this dietary endeavor. When you share a kitchen with people who are not on the gluten-free diet, there can be an increased chance of cross contamination.

Cross contamination can happen when utensils are not thoroughly cleaned before using them for gluten free food. For example, if the same toaster is used to toast gluten free and regular bread, without proper cleaning, cross contamination may occur. Double dipping a crumb coated knife into a common jar of peanut butter or jam can contaminate the condiment, and you may not even realize it! It is important that you let the people you live with know about your dietary restrictions and let them know how important it is for you that they take certain precautions too.

You can also label jars, containers and cutlery using colored tapes to differentiate gluten free foods from the gluten containing foods. This can help in preventing cross contamination.

Chapter 2: The Health Benefits of the Gluten Free Diet

The gluten-free diet has gained a lot of popularity in the recent years. Most people may consider it to be a "fad" that will soon fade, but the fact is that it works for people and it is around to stay for a long, long time.

You can find special sections with all kinds of gluten-free products at most grocery stores; products that were unheard of a few years ago! But, even with its increasing popularity, most people are in the dark about the health benefits one can reap by following the gluten-free diet.

As mentioned before, gluten is a protein that is commonly found in some grains. Gluten is the component of the grain that helps foods retain their elasticity while the food is fermented during production. Gluten is the reason why the bread we eat is not too chewy and other foods do not have a dough like sticky texture.

Why has gluten free shot to the forefront so suddenly and quickly?

Recent years have seen a rise in the number of people suffering from celiac disease or gluten sensitivity. With the gradual increase in cases, the gluten-free diet has come into the limelight, with a lot of physicians and nutritionists studying the diet and its effects on the human body.

The gluten free diet has a lot of benefits for the person following it; from reduced cholesterol in the body, marked increase in energy levels in the body and better digestive health – even if you suffer from gluten intolerance.

When you embark on the gluten free diet, you cut down on a lot of foods in your diet that are generally unhealthy and are the main cause of obesity, such as, fried foods, because most of them are either battered or breaded before frying and most desserts that are rich in fats and sugar because they also need a certain degree of gluten to retain their elasticity.

The benefits of avoiding 'Processed' foods

Most convenience foods available on the market today contain varying quantities of gluten in them and are highly processed, making them extremely unhealthy for you. Some of the reasons why these foods are unhealthy and you are better off avoiding them are as follows:

Processed foods contain a lot of artificial flavors and various chemicals – a lot of chemicals are added to the foods so that they taste good and have a long shelf life.

When you cut all the unhealthy foods from your diet, you are left with select foods that you can actually consume. These are all healthy and nutritious foods, such as fruits and vegetables that provide your body with energy, nutrients and fiber, without having a negative impact on the body.

Healthy foods also provide your body with much-needed antioxidants that help you ward off germs and viruses that can make you extremely ill.

Eliminating gluten from your diet can reduce the pressure on your heart and reduce your chances of contracting cardiovascular diseases, diabetes and other weight related diseases and even certain types of cancer.

Health benefits of going gluten free

The body does not recognize gluten. So when gluten enters the intestines of a person with an autoimmune disease, the body's immunity system attacks it, causing a lot of damage to the body. The digestive tract is unable to extract nutrients from the food, starving the body of nutrients.

Gluten also increases the inflammation in the bodies of people who suffer from inflammatory diseases, such as the Crohn's disease or people who suffer from lupus.

Going gluten free energizes your body, making you feel fresh and healthy. This is because you eat healthier and your body gets a lot more nutrients than it usually gets when your diet consists of junk and processed foods

Autistic children benefit from going gluten free and there is a significant improvement in their symptoms and their overall behavior.

Gluten free is healthy, you just need to be cautious

When you cut off all the unhealthy processed foods, you end up eating "real" unprocessed foods. These foods help in promoting a healthy weight loss cycle and you can even maintain your weight by consuming a well-balanced diet that contains the required quantities of the macros – carbs, proteins and fats.

When you are buying pre-packaged foods or processed foods (such as sauces, condiments, etc.), be sure you read the labels closely. With the FDA guidelines having many loopholes, a lot of foods that do contain small quantities of gluten are being marketed as "gluten free".

While you are keeping a track of labels, also keep a track of the replacements you buy. With the increased popularity of the gluten-free diet, a lot of companies have come up with gluten-free variants of the regular old junk foods and high carb products. You can find gluten-free bread, beers, cakes, pastries, donuts, pizza bread, etc. These foods are usually highly processed and just add empty calories without providing you with any nutrition.

Remember, if you want to lose weight, you need to cut out all those unhealthy foods – just because they are gluten-free, it doesn't make them healthy!

Chapter 3: Case Studies of Gluten Free Diets Working

The regular and typical American diet is making us extremely sick! Consumption of the whole grain and low-fat diet is usually recommended to stay healthy, but it isn't working now, is it? In fact, this diet causes more problems in the body than it corrects.

Yes, some people may see "results" by way of weight loss when they strictly count calories, but let us be honest, this diet is neither easy to follow nor one of the healthiest diets around. Rather, a lot of times, people end up with a vitamin deficiency due to strict calorie control!

Now, on the other hand, the gluten-free diet is a foolproof way to lose weight easily, while staying healthy. It ensures that you get all the nutrients you require while cutting off unhealthy foods from your diet. Here are some of the success stories of celebrities and others, who opted for a healthy living by following the gluten-free diet:

Celebrities:

Celebrities are people too, and despite popular belief, they aren't perfect in any way! Here are 3 celebrities who diligently followed the gluten free diet and lost weight successfully!

Russell Crowe

Russell Crowe is a famous Academy Award-winning Australian actor, who is best known for his portrayal of the Roman General Maximus Decimus Meridius in the historic movie Gladiator (2000). The actor switched to a gluten free diet in 2011, with the intention of getting back into shape.

Russell does not have any gluten intolerance, nor does he suffer from celiac disease. He tweeted that by following the gluten-free diet (& exercising) he lost close to 16 pounds!

David Babaii

You may not have heard of him, but David Babaii is a celebrity hair stylist and has featured as a judge on the second season of "Shear Genius," an American reality show centered on hair styling. His client, Gwyneth Paltrow, a celiac patient and gluten free diet advocate encouraged him to switch to the gluten-free diet.

David does not suffer from celiac disease or any kind of gluten intolerance. The end result was that he lost about 135 pounds by following the gluten-free diet.

Lady Gaga

Back in 2012, the famous pop star put the world's media into a frenzy when she announced to the world that she was going gluten free with the goal of being energized on her international tour and losing 10 pounds.

Commoners:

Hippocrates famously said, "Let food be thy medicine and let medicine be thy food."

You can solve most health issues by modifying your diet and eating well – all you need to do is be patient while your body adjusts to the change in your diet. Here are the success stories of few people who battled illnesses and changed their lives around by going gluten free. (Their names have been changed to protect their identities)

Deborah Potter

At the age of 35, Deborah had experienced 4 miscarriages while attempting to conceive another baby. With her biological clock ticking rather loudly, she also suspected that she had thyroid issues and hormonal imbalance. Her goal was to lose about 15 to 17 pounds and feel more energized, in order to keep up with her children, while planning another one. With young children, she wanted a solution that could be easily implemented family wide, without any issues.

She was prescribed a simple gluten free diet that accommodated the fact that she wasn't a great cook. Her husband and children initially found it difficult to adjust to the change, but they quickly caught on. Within a month Deborah lost about 10 pounds, her husband's blood pressure was back to normal (he had a high blood pressure problem) and her children were less irritable.

Within another few weeks, she was able to conceive. She followed the prescribed lifestyle through her pregnancy (with a few tweaks) and gave birth to a healthy baby boy.

Andrew Johnson

Andrew, a 27-year-old media professional was tall, but his impressive physique was marred by the fact that he was a good 100 pounds overweight. He maintained that he found it extremely difficult to stick to a particular diet plan and when he had a craving, he had to satiate it. Along with losing weight, his goal was to build more muscle and get a leaner physique. His diet then was full of processed foods, and he cited that his busy schedule left him not much time to cook for himself. His unhealthy diet had resulted in skin issues, digestive troubles and light insomnia.

Fed up with how his irregular eating habits were affecting his physical and mental health, he decided to switch to a gluten-free diet. Initially, he found it a bit difficult to adjust and felt really awkward at team lunches or client meetings that involved food, but with his dedication, he lost more than 20 pounds in the first month of his lifestyle change. By the end of the second month, he lost a cumulative 40 pounds and noticed a great difference in his skin, digestion, sleep and mental issues. He even ended up trading in his sedentary lifestyle for a more active lifestyle that included plenty of exercising.

By the end of 6 months, he not only reached his target weight, but he was also slowly working his way towards achieving the lean muscular physique that he wished for.

Matthew Riddle

With a family history of every possible disease, 52-year-old Matthew was not looking good. With severe digestive and skin issues that had plagued him for a better part of 20 years, his issues were getting worse with his age, increasing his anxiety and blood pressure from the fear of contracting the hereditary diseases. He also had high cholesterol and was a borderline pre-diabetic.

Add to this, some of his favorite foods were: bread, donuts, coffee, pastries, rolls, soda, pancakes, chips, etc.

Matthew was firm in his stance that any lifestyle change he was expected to undergo could not cut any of his favorite foods from his diet. He disliked most vegetables consumed by man, and whenever he consumed any proteins, he needed to have them with bread.

If not for the constant nagging of his wife, he would have been a diabetic with high blood pressure and high cholesterol by now.

But, once he promised her he would try to change his lifestyle and eat healthily, he stuck to it and agreed that he would try the gluten free diet for 2 months, and only 2 months, not a day more.

By the time two months ended, Matthew had lost a good 42 pounds, his skin was glowing and his digestive issues were not as troublesome as before. He mentioned that at the end of two months his wife presented him with a buffet of all his old favorite foods as a reward, but he felt terrible about eating them and ended up not eating any of them!

Matthew is dedicated to the gluten-free diet, and now at the age of 60, he is still continuing with the diet. His digestion issues are long gone and his doctor has told him that his heart looks really young for his age.

So, here were some cases where people – celebrities and commoners alike - overcame a lot of mental and physical issues, while losing weight, by following the gluten-free diet. For best results, it is advisable that you consult your doctor or a trained nutritionist before switching diets.

Chapter 4: Foods to Eat and Foods to Avoid

Foods You Can Consume

Gluten is mainly found in grains. Once you look past them you will realize that a lot of delicious and healthy foods do not have any gluten in them. Listed here are the foods that you can consume:

- ✓ Unprocessed beans, nuts and seeds in their natural form, such as garbanzo beans, pumpkin seeds, peanuts, walnuts, kidney beans, sunflower seeds, to name a few.
- ✓ Grass fed meats (beef, venison, lamb, etc.) wild caught fresh fish (salmon, tuna, sea bass, etc.), seafood (shrimp, crab, etc.) and fresh poultry (chicken, turkey, etc.) – without any batter, marinade or bread coating.
- ✓ Vegetables and fruits, such as apples, carrots, beetroots, strawberries, lemons, coconuts, etc.
- ✓ Almost all dairy products (grass fed) (check labels to see that no grains are used as preservatives or additives), such as cheese, cottage cheese, etc.

While most grains have gluten in them, some grains are truly gluten free and can be consumed freely, such as:

- Amaranth
- Buckwheat
- Arrowroot
- Corn and cornmeal
- Gluten free flours (rice, corn, bean, soy, potato)
- Flax
- Hominy (corn)
- Quinoa
- Millet
- Rice
- Soy
- Sorghum
- Teff
- Tapioca

Foods You Need To Completely Avoid

All the foods that contain even tiny amounts of these ingredients contain gluten and should be avoided at all costs (especially if you suffer from celiac disease or gluten intolerance):

- Barley
- Triticale (a hybrid cross between rye and wheat)
- Rye
- Wheat

Avoiding wheat can be extremely difficult because the product is marketed under various names and it can be difficult to keep a track of all its variants. You can understand the versatility of wheat by just walking through the flour section of your supermarket and checking out the various kinds of wheat flour available, making it difficult to keep track. Here are some products and ingredients that you should avoid:

- Durum flour
- Graham flour
- Farina
- Kamut or oriental wheat or Khorasan wheat
- Spelt
- Semolina

Foods You Should Avoid Unless Labeled "Gluten Free"

These are the foods that usually contain gluten, but now have gluten-free variants available in the market. Read the labels and only consume them if they are either labeled gluten free or are made using corn, soy, rice or other gluten-free grains:

- Beer
- Cakes and pies (only pie crust or filled pies)
- Breads
- Candies
- Communion wafers
- Cereals
- Croutons
- Cookies and crackers
- French-fries
- Imitation meat, poultry or seafood

- Gravies (ready to eat or powdered)
- Matzo (Jewish flatbread)
- Processed meats (processed cold cuts, dried meats, jerky, etc.)
- Pastas
- Salad dressings
- Seasoned rice mixes
- Sauces, including soy sauce, hoisin sauce, etc.
- Seasoned junk food
- Soups and soup bases
- Self-basting poultry
- Vegetables in sauce

Certain grains, such as oats, are usually grown alongside wheat and may get contaminated with gluten during the growth or processing stages. For this very reason, most dieticians and doctors advise that oats should be avoided unless specifically labeled to be gluten free.

You should also keep track of certain products that may not specifically contain the words gluten free on their label. This includes:

- Any medicines that may use a gluten based binding agent
- Any food additives that may contain modified starch or malt flavoring

Chapter 5: Gluten Free Appetizers & Snacks Recipes

Refreshing Fresh Tomato Salsa

Serves: 2

Ingredients

- 1 large tomato, chopped
- 2 1/2 Serrano chilies, finely chopped
- 1/4 cup finely diced onion
- 1/4 cup chopped fresh cilantro
- 1 teaspoon lime juice
- 1/2 teaspoon salt

Directions

1. Place the chopped tomato and onion in a medium sized mixing bowl.

2. Add in the Serrano chilies, cilantro, lime juice and salt.

3. Mix well until well combined.

4. Cover the bowl using a plastic wrap and chill in the refrigerator for at least an hour or two.

5. Serve with a side of carrot sticks or beetroot sticks.

6. Enjoy!

BLT Style Dip

Serves: 8

Ingredients

- 1/2 pound bacon
- 1/2 cup sour cream
- 1/2 cup mayonnaise
- 1/2 tomato, carefully peeled, seeds removed and diced finely

Directions

1. Heat a large deep skillet over a medium flame. Add in the bacon and heat until the bacon is well browned and crispy.

2. Once done, remove the bacon from the skillet and place on paper towels to drain the excess fat from it.

3. Place the mayonnaise in a medium sized mixing bowl. Add in the sour cream and mix well until well combined.

4. Gently crumble the bacon using your hands and add to the mayonnaise and sour cream mix.

5. Add in the tomatoes just before serving.

6. Serve immediately.

7. Enjoy!

Delicious Ham and Cream Cheese Roll Ups with Dill Pickle

Serves: 10

Ingredients

- 10 slices cooked ham
- 10 dill pickle spears
- 2 (8 ounce) packages cream cheese, softened

Directions

1. Separate the ham slices and lay them on a kitchen towel. Make sure they do not overlap. Using another kitchen towel pat until dry.

2. Spoon about a tablespoon of cream cheese on a slice of ham, spreading it in an even layer. Repeat with the remaining ham slices.

3. Place a dill pickle spear on one end of the cream cheese covered ham slice, about half an inch away from the edge.

4. Gently roll the ham over the dill pickle to make a small cylinder. Secure it in place with a toothpick.

5. Serve immediately or chilled, as per your preference.

6. Enjoy!

Quick and Easy Guacamole

Serves: 8

Ingredients

- 1 avocado
- 1/2 clove garlic, minced
- 1/2 small onion, finely chopped
- 1/2 ripe tomato, chopped
- Salt, to taste
- 1/2 lime, juiced
- Freshly ground black pepper, to taste

Directions

1. Scoop out the fleshy part of the avocado using a spoon and place it in a serving bowl.

2. Using the back of a spoon or a potato masher, mash the avocado pulp until smooth.

3. Add in the onion, tomato, salt, garlic, lime juice and pepper. Mix well until well combined.

4. Taste and add in more seasoning or lime juice if required.

5. Cover the bowl with some plastic wrap and let the guacamole chill in the fridge for a few hours.

6. Serve chilled with some carrot sticks or beetroot sticks.

7. Enjoy!

Buffalo Chicken Wings

Serves: 4

Ingredients

- 2 cups vegetable oil for deep frying
- 2 tablespoons butter
- 12 chicken wings, wings cut into two halves at the joint and the tips removed
- 1 1/2 teaspoons distilled white vinegar
- Salt, to taste
- 7 1/2 teaspoons hot pepper sauce
- Freshly ground black pepper, to taste

Directions

1. Pour the oil into a deep fryer or in a large skillet. Heat the oil to about 375 degrees Fahrenheit (about 190 degrees Celsius).

2. Add the chicken wings slowly and carefully into the hot oil and let them fry for about 10 to 12 minutes.

3. Remove the chicken from the oil and place on paper towels to drain the excess oil.

4. Place the butter in a large skillet and heat on a medium flame until the butter is completely melted.

5. Add the hot pepper sauce and vinegar to the butter and mix well. Add in salt and pepper.

6. Add the prepared chicken to the skillet and cook over a medium to low flame until the chicken pieces are well coated by the sauce. The longer you cook the juicier and tastier your chicken pieces will be.

7. Serve hot.

8. Enjoy!

Creamy and Tangy Cilantro Sauce

Serves: 4

Ingredients

- 1 (8 ounce) package cream cheese, softened
- 1 (7 ounce) can tomatillo salsa
- 1 tablespoon sour cream
- 1 teaspoon freshly ground black pepper
- 1/2 teaspoon ground cumin
- 1 teaspoon celery salt
- 2 teaspoons garlic powder
- 1 tablespoon fresh lime juice
- 1 bunch fresh cilantro, chopped

Directions

1. Place the cream cheese in the jar of a blender or food processor. Add in the sour cream and tomatillo salsa. Blitz until it has a smooth and creamy consistency.

2. Add in the cilantro and blitz again until smooth.

3. Sprinkle in the ground black pepper, ground cumin, celery salt, and garlic powder. Blitz until combined.

4. Pour in the lemon juice and blitz one final time.

5. Use a spatula to empty the contents of the jar into a bowl.

6. Cover the bowl with a plastic wrap and chill the sauce in the refrigerator for a few hours.

7. Serve with your favorite gluten free crackers.

8. Enjoy!

Traditional Hummus

Serves: 8

Ingredients

- 1 cup canned garbanzo beans, liquid drained
- 2 tablespoons lemon juice
- 8 teaspoons tahini
- 1/2 teaspoon salt
- 1 1/2 teaspoons olive oil
- 1 clove garlic, halved
- 1/2 teaspoon minced fresh parsley
- 1/2 pinch paprika

Directions

1. Place the garbanzo beans in the jar of a blender or a food processor and blend until they are smooth and have a paste like consistency.

2. Add in the lemon juice, tahini, salt and garlic to the garbanzo bean paste and blend again until all the *ingredients* are well incorporated.

3. Spoon the prepared mixture into a serving bowl.

4. Lightly pour the olive oil over the prepared mixture, ensuring that the oil doesn't sink in. Sprinkle the parsley and paprika over the oil.

5. Serve immediately with a side of gluten free pita bread.

6. Enjoy!

Gluten Free Artichoke and Spinach Dip

Serves: 3

Ingredients

- 1/2 (14 ounce) can artichoke hearts, liquid drained and coarsely chopped
- 1/2 cup mayonnaise
- 1/2 (10 ounce) package frozen chopped spinach, well thawed and liquid drained
- 1 1/4 cups shredded Monterey Jack cheese, separated
- 1/2 cup grated Parmesan cheese

Directions

1. Crank up your oven to about 350 degrees Fahrenheit (about 175 degrees Celsius) and let it preheat for about 20 minutes or so.

2. Pour some oil in a 1-pint (1/2 quart) baking dish and lightly spread the oil into all the corners using a tissue.

3. Place the chopped artichoke hearts in a medium sized mixing bowl.

4. Add the mayonnaise, spinach, Parmesan cheese and about 1 cup of the Monterey Jack cheese to the artichoke hearts.

5. Mix well until well combined.

6. Spoon the prepared mixture into the greased baking dish and gently press using the back of the spoon to ensure there are no air bubbles.

7. Cover the dip with the remaining ¼ cup of Monterey Jack cheese.

8. Pop the baking dish into the preheated oven and bake for about 15 to 20 minutes or until the cheese has completely melted.

9. Serve hot.

10. Enjoy!

Buttery and Tangy Grilled Basil Shrimp

Serves: 4

Ingredients

- 3 and 1/4 teaspoons olive oil
- 1 lemon, juiced
- 8 and 1/4 teaspoons butter, melted
- 4 teaspoons Dijon mustard
- 2 cloves garlic, minced
- 10 3/4 teaspoons minced fresh basil leaves
- Salt, to taste
- 1 1/4 pounds fresh shrimp, shells and vein removed
- Freshly ground white pepper, to taste

Directions

1. Pour the olive oil and butter together into a shallow and non-porous dish.

2. Pour in the lemon juice and mix well until well incorporated.

3. Add in the mustard, garlic and basil and mix well. Season to taste with the salt and white pepper.

4. Add the shrimp to the bowl and toss well until well coated.

5. Cover the dish with a plastic wrap and refrigerate for an hour or two, so that the shrimp can soak up the marinade.

6. Preheat the grill for about 20 minutes on the high setting.

7. Drain the shrimp from the marinade and thread them onto the skewers. Keep the size of your grill in mind so that you don't end up threading too many on a single skewer. If using wooden or bamboo skewers, soak them for about half an hour in warm water before using.

8. Use a pastry brush to lightly oil the grate and place the skewers on the grill.

9. Cook the skewers for about 2 to 3 minutes on each side or until the shrimp become opaque.

10. Serve hot with your favorite gluten free condiment and a side of grilled vegetables.

11. Enjoy!

Grilled Marinated Shrimp

Serves: 3

Ingredients

- 1/2 cup olive oil
- 1/2 lemon, juiced
- 2 tablespoons chopped fresh parsley
- 1 tablespoon hot pepper sauce
- 1 1/2 teaspoons tomato paste
- 1 1/2 cloves garlic, minced
- 1 teaspoon dried oregano
- 1/2 teaspoon ground black pepper
- 1/2 teaspoon salt
- 1 pound large shrimp, shell and vein removed, but tail attached

Directions

1. Combine the olive oil, lemon juice, garlic, oregano, black pepper, parsley, hot sauce, tomato paste and salt together in a mixing bowl. Whisk well until all the *ingredients* are well combined.

2. Spoon about 2 to 3 tablespoons of the mixture into a small mixing bowl and set aside. This will be used for basting.

3. Add the shrimp to a large re-sealable bag. Pour in the leftover marinade and seal the bag. Shake well until the marinade coats the shrimp. Refrigerate for about 3 to 4 hours.

4. If you do not have a re-sealable plastic bag, you can marinate the shrimp in a bowl too – just remember to cover the bowl with some plastic wrap before refrigerating.

5. Preheat the grill for about 20 minutes on the medium low heat.

6. Drain the shrimp from the marinade and thread them onto the skewers, piercing once near the head and once near the tail. Keep the size of your grill in mind so that you don't end up threading too many on a single skewer. If using wooden or bamboo skewers, soak them for about half an hour in warm water before using.

7. Use a pastry brush to lightly oil the grate and place the skewers on the grill.

8. Cook the shrimp for about 5 to 7 minutes per side or until the shrimp turn opaque. Make sure to frequently baste the shrimp with the reserved marinade, as this will ensure that the shrimp is juicy and full of moisture.

9. Serve hot with your favorite gluten free condiment and a side of grilled vegetables.

10. Enjoy

Healthy Baked Kale Chips

Serves: 3

Ingredients

- 1/2 bunch kale
- 1/2 teaspoon seasoned salt
- 1 1/2 teaspoons olive oil

Directions

1. Crank up your oven to 350 degrees Fahrenheit (about 175 degrees Celsius) and let it preheat for about 20 minutes. Rub some oil over a cookie sheet and then cover it with some parchment paper. This will ensure that the parchment paper doesn't move around while cooking.

2. Use some kitchen scissors or a knife to separate the leaves from the stem.

3. Cut the kale leaves into bite sized pieces and wash well to remove all the dirt and grit from them. You can also use a salad spinner to wash them.

4. Dry the kale leaves on a kitchen towel to rid them of the excess moisture.

5. Transfer the kale to a large mixing bowl and add in the olive oil. Sprinkle the salt over the kale and toss them well until they are well coated by the oil.

6. Spread the kale on the parchment paper lined cookie sheet in a single layer.

7. Pop into the preheated oven and bake for about 12 to 17 minutes or until the edges of the kale are lightly browned.

8. Cool before serving.

9. Enjoy!

Spiced Pumpkin Seeds

Serves: 4

Ingredients

- 2 1/4 teaspoons margarine, melted
- 1/8 teaspoon garlic salt
- 1/4 teaspoon salt
- 1 cup raw whole pumpkin seeds
- 1 teaspoon Worcestershire sauce

Directions

1. Crank up your oven to 275 degrees Fahrenheit (about 135 degrees Celsius) and let it preheat for about 20 minutes. Rub some oil over a cookie sheet and then cover it with some parchment paper. This will ensure that the parchment paper doesn't move around while cooking.

2. In a small mixing bowl, combine the margarine, garlic salt, salt and Worcestershire sauce together. Whisk well until all the *ingredients* are well combined.

3. Place the pumpkin seeds in a medium sized mixing bowl. Pour the prepared condiment mix over the pumpkin seeds. Toss well until the pumpkin seeds are well coated.

4. Spread the pumpkin seeds in an even layer on the parchment lined cookie sheet.

5. Bake for about 60 to 70 minutes, stirring the seeds around every 20 minutes.

6. Cool and serve.

7. Enjoy!

Chapter 6: Breakfast and Brunch Recipes

Eggs with Zucchini

Serves: 2

Ingredients

- 4 teaspoons olive oil
- 2 small zucchinis, thinly sliced
- Salt, to taste
- 2 eggs, well beaten and bubbly
- Freshly ground black pepper, to taste

Directions

1. Pour the oil into a small skillet and heat over a medium low flame.
2. Once the oil is lightly smoking, add the sliced zucchini to the pan and sauté until the zucchini is tender.
3. Spread the sautéed zucchini into an even layer in the pan.
4. Add the seasoning to the eggs and pour the eggs over the zucchini.
5. Cook until the egg is firm and not jiggling.
6. Serve hot with some freshly squeezed orange juice on the side.
7. Enjoy!

Delicious and Healthy Gluten Free Pancakes

Serves: 5

Ingredients

- 1/2 cup rice flour
- 8 teaspoons potato starch
- 4 1/2 teaspoons tapioca flour
- 2 tablespoons dry buttermilk powder
- 3/4 teaspoon baking powder
- 1/2 packet sugar substitute
- 1/4 teaspoon baking soda
- 1/4 teaspoon xanthan gum
- 1/4 teaspoon salt
- 1 egg
- 1 cup water
- 4 1/2 teaspoons canola oil

Directions

1. Sieve together the rice flour, potato starch, sugar substitute, baking soda, xanthan gum, tapioca flour, dry buttermilk powder, baking powder and salt together in the large mixing bowl.

2. In another small mixing bowl, whisk together the eggs, oil and water together.

3. Pour the wet *ingredients* into the flour mix and mix well until well blended. If there are a few lumps, don't worry.

4. Pour some oil into a large griddle or skillet and heat over a medium high flame.

5. Slowly spoon about half cup of the batter onto the hot skillet and cook until there are small bubbles on the surface of the pancake.

6. Flip the pancake over and cook until the other side is well browned.

7. Repeat with the remaining batter.

8. Serve hot, topped with some pure maple syrup and a few blueberries or raspberries.

9. Enjoy!

Gluten Free Ham and Cheese Breakfast Quiche

Serves: 10

Ingredients

- 4 (12 ounce) packages frozen hash brown potatoes, thawed and drained
- 2 cups cooked diced ham
- 2/3 cup butter, melted
- 2 cups shredded Monterey Jack cheese
- 1 cup heavy whipping cream
- 4 eggs

Directions

1. Crank up your oven to 425 degrees Fahrenheit (about 220 degrees Celsius) and let it preheat for about 20 minutes.

2. Squeeze the hash brown potatoes well to remove the extra moisture that may be present in the potatoes.

3. Place the potatoes in a mixing bowl and pour the butter over them. Mix well until well combined.

4. Transfer the potatoes into an ungreased 10-inch baking dish. Gently press the potato and butter mixture until it covers the bottom and sides of the pan.

5. Pop the baking dish into the preheated oven and bake for about 25 to 30 minutes or until the potato mix is golden brown.

6. Carefully remove the pan from the oven and let it cool a bit.

7. Place the ham in a single layer over the potato layer and cover it with the cheese.

8. In a medium sized mixing bowl combine together the cream and the eggs and whisk well until well combined.

9. Pour the egg and cream mix over the cheese layer.

10. Pop the baking dish back into the oven and continue baking it at 425 degrees Fahrenheit (about 220 degrees Celsius) for about 40 minutes or until the quiche is well set.

11. Remove from the oven and cool the quiche in the pan for about 5 to 7 minutes before removing it from the pan.

12. Serve immediately.

13. Enjoy!

Quick Greek Style Scrambled Eggs

Serves: 1

Ingredients

- 1 1/2 teaspoons butter
- 1/2 teaspoon water
- 1 1/2 eggs
- Salt, to taste
- 1/4 cup crumbled feta cheese
- Freshly ground black pepper, to taste

Directions

1. Place the butter in a skillet and melt it over a medium high flame.
2. While the butter gets heated, add the eggs to a medium sized bowl.
3. Add in the water and whisk well until well combined.
4. Pour the eggs into the hot skillet and add in the crumbled feta cheese.
5. Stir the egg mixture occasionally to scramble it.
6. Season to taste with salt and pepper.
7. Serve hot with a side of some hash browns and fresh fruit juice.
8. Enjoy!

Baby Spinach Omelet

Serves: 2

Ingredients

- 4 eggs
- 3 tablespoons grated Parmesan cheese
- 2 cups torn baby spinach leaves
- 1/2 teaspoon onion powder
- Salt, to taste
- 1/4 teaspoon ground nutmeg
- Freshly ground black pepper, to taste

Directions

1. Place the eggs in a medium sized mixing bowl and whisk well.

2. Add the Parmesan cheese and baby spinach to the eggs and whisk well.

3. Add in the nutmeg, black pepper, onion powder and salt and whisk well.

4. Coat a medium sized skillet with some cooking spray and heat over a medium high flame until lightly smoking.

5. Add the egg mixture to the skillet and cook for about 3 to 5 minutes or until the eggs are semi set.

6. Carefully, using a spatula, flip the eggs over and continue cooking on a medium high flame for about 2 to 3 minutes.

7. Turn the heat down to a low and cover and cook for another minute or two or until the egg reaches the desired degree of doneness.

8. Serve hot with some toasted gluten free bread on the side.

9. Enjoy!

Sautéed Cinnamon Apples

Serves: 4

Ingredients

- 2 tablespoons butter
- 2 large tart apples – peel and core removed, cut into ¼ inch thick slices
- 1 teaspoon cornstarch
- 1/4 cup brown sugar
- 1/4 cup cold water
- 1/4 teaspoon ground cinnamon

Directions

1. Place the butter in a large saucepan or skillet and melt the butter over a medium high flame.

2. Once the butter has melted, add the apple slices to the pan.

3. Cook for about 7 to 10 minutes or until the apples are tender, but not very mushy. While the apples cook, make sure you constantly stir them around or they will stick to the bottom of the pan.

4. Add some water to the cornstarch and mix well until dissolved.

5. Pour the cornstarch mix into the pan and mix well until the apples are well coated.

6. Add the cinnamon and brown sugar to the apple and continue heating on a high flame for about 2 to 3 minutes, while constantly stirring the mixture around.

7. Remove the apples from the pan and serve them warm.

8. Enjoy!

Country Style Fried Potatoes

Serves: 3

Ingredients

- 8 teaspoons shortening
- 1/2 teaspoon salt
- 3 large potatoes, peel removed and cut into cubes
- 1/4 teaspoon ground black pepper
- 1/4 teaspoon paprika
- 1/4 teaspoon garlic powder

Directions

1. Place the shortening in a large cast iron skillet and heat it over a medium high flame. Once the shortening has melted, add the potatoes to the pan and cook them until golden brown, while constantly stirring them around.

2. Once done, transfer the potatoes to a large mixing bowl.

3. Add in the salt, garlic powder, pepper and paprika. Toss well until well-seasoned.

4. Serve hot as a side with some bacon and eggs.

5. Enjoy

Healthy Corned Beef Hash

Serves: 3

Ingredients

- 3 large potatoes, peel removed and finely diced
- 1/2 medium onion, chopped
- 1/2 (12 ounce) can corned beef, cut into bite sized chunks
- 1/2 cup beef broth

Directions

1. Heat a large deep skillet over a medium high flame.

2. Add the potatoes, onion, corned beef and beef broth to the pan.

3. Cover the skillet and let the contents simmer in the beef broth until the potatoes are soft and mushy.

4. Mix well and serve immediately.

5. Enjoy!

Oven Roasted Rosemary Butter New Potato Wedges

Serves: 2

Ingredients

- 3/4 pound new potatoes, cut into large wedges
- 1 teaspoon fresh rosemary
- 2 tablespoons butter
- Freshly ground black pepper, to taste
- Salt, to taste

Directions

1. Crank up your oven to 450 degrees Fahrenheit (about 230 degrees Celsius) and let it preheat for about 20 minutes.

2. Place the butter in a small skillet and heat over a medium high flame until melted.

3. Add the rosemary, pepper and salt to the melted butter and mix well.

4. Place the potato wedges in a large mixing bowl and pour the seasoned butter over the potato wedges.

5. Toss well until all the potatoes are well coated.

6. Place the potatoes in a single layer in a baking dish.

7. Pop the baking dish into the preheated oven and bake for about 25 to 30 minutes or until golden brown, stopping the oven every 7 minutes or so to toss the potatoes to ensure even cooking.

8. Serve hot with some bacon and eggs.

9. Enjoy!

Scrambled Feta Eggs

Serves: 2

Ingredients

- 1 1/2 teaspoons butter
- 2 eggs, beaten
- 2 tablespoons chopped onion
- 2 tablespoons chopped tomatoes
- Salt
- 1 tablespoon crumbled feta cheese
- Freshly ground black pepper, to taste

Directions

1. Place the butter in a small skillet. Heat the skillet over a medium flame, until the butter has melted.

2. Add the onions to the butter and sauté until the onions are tender and translucent. This should take about4 to 5 minutes.

3. Pour the beaten eggs over the onion and cook them for about 5 minutes.

4. Stir the eggs around occasionally to scramble them.

5. Once the eggs are almost done, add in the feta cheese and tomatoes.

6. Season to taste with salt and pepper.

7. Continue cooking until the cheese melts.

8. Serve hot over some toasted gluten free bread.

9. Enjoy!

Chapter 7: Meal Recipes

Gluten Free Shrimp Creole

Serves: 3

Ingredients

- 1 1/2 pounds medium shrimp – shells and vein removed, shells reserved
- 1/2 carrot, finely chopped
- 1/4 onion, chopped
- 1 strip celery, chopped
- 8 teaspoons bacon grease
- 2 cups water
- 1 onion, chopped
- 1 1/2 teaspoons minced garlic
- 1 strip celery, chopped
- 1/2 large chopped green bell pepper
- Salt, to taste
- 1 bay leaves
- 3/4 teaspoon freshly ground black pepper
- 1/2 teaspoon cayenne pepper
- 1 teaspoon brown sugar
- 1/2 teaspoon hot pepper sauce or according to taste
- 1/2 teaspoon dried thyme
- 1/2 teaspoon dried rosemary
- 1/2 teaspoon dried basil
- 1 cup canned tomato sauce
- 2 tomatoes, chopped
- 1/2 cup chopped green onion

Directions

1. Place the reserved shrimp shells in a medium sized stockpot. Add in the ¼ onion, ½ carrot, 1 celery strip and 2 cups water.

2. Heat over a medium high flame and let the liquid simmer for about 1 hour, stirring every 10 minutes. Simmer the liquid uncovered.

3. Strain the prepared broth and add the liquid to a small saucepan. Heat the saucepan over a high flame until the liquid is reduced to about 1 cup. Take the pan off heat

and set aside.

4. Place the grease in a heavy bottomed skillet and heat over a medium high flame.

5. Add the onions, garlic, celery and green bell pepper to the pan. Cook until the vegetables soften and begin to brown around the edges.

6. Add in the bay leaves, ground black pepper, cayenne pepper, 1 cup prepared shrimp stock, salt, brown sugar and hot sauce to the pan.

7. Heat until lightly bubbling.

8. Once the mix is boiling, add in the crushed rosemary, crushed basil, tomato sauce, crushed thyme and tomatoes to the pan.

9. Cover the pan and reduce the heat to a medium low. Let the liquid simmer for an hour, stirring the mix around occasionally.

10. Add the cleaned shrimp to the pan and mix well.

11. Take the pan of heat and cover it.

12. Set the pan aside for about 20 to 25 minutes until the shrimp becomes pink.

13. Add a sprinkling of green onion on the top.

14. Serve hot over a bed of steamed rice.

15. Enjoy!

Baked Egg and Veggie Pie

Serves: 4

Ingredients

- 1/2 large baking potato
- 1/2 teaspoon salt
- 3 eggs
- 1/4 teaspoon ground black pepper
- 1 tablespoon olive oil
- 2 tablespoons chopped fresh parsley
- 1/2 onion, chopped
- 2 tablespoons chopped fresh mushrooms
- 2 tablespoons chopped red bell pepper
- 1/4 cup chopped ham
- 2 tablespoons shredded Cheddar cheese
- 1/2 tomato, sliced

Directions

1. Salt a medium pot of water and heat over a high flame until bubbling.
2. Add the potatoes to the salted water and cook for about 15 to 20 minutes or until the potatoes are tender, but still firm.
3. Drain the potatoes from the water and cool completely before peeling. Cut into thin slices and set aside.
4. Crank up the oven to 350 degrees Fahrenheit (about 175 degrees Celsius) and let it preheat for about 20 minutes.
5. Place the eggs in a medium sized mixing bowl and add in the salt, parsley and pepper. Whisk well until well combined.
6. Pour the olive oil into a cast iron skillet and heat over a medium high flame.
7. Once the oil is lightly smoking, add in the onion and red bell pepper. Cook until softened.
8. Add in the mushrooms and continue cooking.
9. Once the mushrooms start shrinking, ad in the potato slices, chopped ham and tomato slices to the pan.
10. Add in the prepared egg mixture and mix gently until well combined.
11. Take the pan off heat and sprinkle the cheese over the mixture.
12. Pop the skillet into the preheated oven and bake for about 15 to 20 minutes or until the eggs are firm.
13. Cool for a few minutes before cutting out slices and serving.
14. Enjoy!

Grilled Teriyaki Flank Steak

Serves: 2

Ingredients

- 1/4 cup wine
- 2 tablespoons olive oil
- 1/4 cup soy sauce
- 2 tablespoons brown sugar
- 1 clove garlic, crushed
- 2 tablespoons grated fresh ginger root
- 3/4 pound beef flank steak
- 1/2 teaspoon ground black pepper

Directions

1. Combine the olive oil, soy sauce, and wine together in a medium sized mixing bowl. Whisk well until all the *ingredients* are well combined.

2. Add in the brown sugar, crushed garlic, grated ginger and pepper to the mixing bowl and mix well.

3. Place the flank steak in a large re-sealable plastic bag. Pour the prepared marinade over the steak and seal the bag. Toss the bag until the steak is well coated by the marinade.

4. Refrigerate the steak for about 8 hours or overnight if possible.

5. Preheat the grill on a medium high heat for about 10 minutes.

6. Drain the steak from the marinade and discard the extra marinade.

7. Place the marinated steak on the preheated grill and cook for about 7 to 9 minutes per side or as per your desired degree of doneness.

8. For a rare cooked steak the internal temperature of the steak should be at least 145 degrees Fahrenheit (about 63 degrees Celsius).

9. Once done, take the steak off the grill and let it rest for about 5 minutes.

10. Slice the beef against the grain and serve with some grilled vegetables on the side.

11. Enjoy!

Easy Grilled Chicken Breast with Grilled Vegetables and Bacon

Serves: 2

Ingredients

- 1/2 pound peppered bacon
- 1 1/2 medium carrots, peeled and chopped
- 1 1/2 medium potatoes, chopped
- 1/2 medium onion, chopped
- 1/4 cup butter
- Garlic salt, to taste
- 2 chicken breast halves, skinless and boneless

Directions

1. Place the bacon in a heavy bottomed skillet and heat over a medium high flame, until the bacon is well browned. Drain the bacon from the fat and place on a kitchen towel for further draining. Chop the bacon roughly and keep it aside.

2. Cut out 2 large squares out of heavy-duty aluminum foil.

3. Divide the potatoes, onion and carrots in two equal portions and place them in the center of each foil square.

4. Place one chicken breast on each vegetable pile.

5. Top the chicken breast with the chopped bacon.

6. Add about 2 tablespoons of butter over the bacon and sprinkle garlic salt over it.

7. Carefully fold the aluminum foil to make a tightly sealed packet.

8. Preheat a grill on a medium high setting or about 10 minutes.

9. Place the prepared packet on the grill and cook for about 20 to 25 minutes or until the juices run clear and the chicken is no longer pink.

10. Serve hot.

11. Enjoy!

Buttery Grilled Sea Bass

Serves: 3

Ingredients

- 1/8 teaspoon garlic powder
- 1/8 teaspoon paprika
- 1/8 teaspoon onion powder
- Lemon pepper to taste
- 1 pound sea bass
- Sea salt to taste
- 4 1/2 teaspoons butter
- 1 1/2 teaspoons chopped Italian flat leaf parsley
- 1 large clove garlic, chopped
- 2 1/4 teaspoons extra virgin olive oil

Directions

1. Preheat the grill on the high heat setting for about 10 to 15 minutes.

2. Combine the garlic powder, paprika, onion powder, and sea salt and lemon pepper together in a small mixing bowl. Mix well.

3. Sprinkle the prepared seasoning over the sea bass and gently rub it in on both sides of the filets.

4. Add the butter to a small saucepan and heat over a medium high flame. Add in the garlic and parsley and continue heating until the butter melts. Take off heat and set aside.

5. Lightly brush some oil over the grate of the grill. Place the fish over the heated grate and cook for about 5 to 7 minutes.

6. Flip the fish over and lightly brush the prepared herb butter over the fish.

7. Continue cooking for another 5 to 7 minutes or until the fish easily flakes when flaked with a fork.

8. Pour some olive oil over the fish and serve immediately with a side of grilled or stir fried vegetables.

9. Enjoy!

Gluten Free Whole Roasted Chicken

Serves: 3

Ingredients

- 1 (1-1/2 pound) whole chicken, giblets removed
- Freshly ground black pepper, to taste
- Salt, to taste
- 1 1/2 teaspoons onion powder, or to taste
- 1/2 stalk celery, leaves removed
- 1/4 cup margarine, divided

Directions

1. Crank up your oven to 350 degrees Fahrenheit (about 175 degrees Celsius) and let the oven preheat for about 20 minutes.

2. Place the whole chicken in a roasting pan. Sprinkle generous amounts of salt and pepper over it and rub the salt onto the chicken on the outside as well as on the inside.

3. Sprinkle the onion powder inside and rub it in using your fingers too.

4. Place about 1-½ tablespoons of the margarine in the cavity of the chicken and place the remaining margarine around the exterior of the chicken in 1-tablespoon dollops.

5. Roughly chop the celery stalk into 2 to 3 large chunks and place it inside the chicken cavity.

6. Pop the baking dish into the preheated oven and bake for about 1 hour and 20 to 25 minutes or until the internal temperature of the chicken reads a minimum of 180 degrees Fahrenheit (82 degrees Celsius).

7. Remove the roasting pan from the oven and baste the chicken with the drippings and margarine.

8. Cover the pan with a large piece of aluminum foil and set aside for about 30 minutes before carving.

9. Serve hot.

10. Enjoy!

Gluten Free Cheese and Herb Pizza Crust

Serves: 4

Ingredients

- 6 tablespoons gluten-free all-purpose baking flour
- 2 tablespoons cornstarch
- 6 1/2 teaspoon garbanzo bean flour
- 2 tablespoons tapioca starch
- 3/4 teaspoon baking powder
- 2 tablespoons grated Parmesan cheese
- 1/2 teaspoon xanthan gum
- 1/2 teaspoon dried oregano
- 1/2 teaspoon Italian seasoning
- 1/4 teaspoon salt
- 1/2 cup lukewarm water
- 1/2 teaspoon white sugar
- 1/2 (.25 ounce) package active dry yeast
- 3/4 teaspoon olive oil
- 1/2 eggs
- 1/4 teaspoon apple cider vinegar
- 1/2 teaspoon white sugar

Directions

1. Crank up your oven to 425 degrees Fahrenheit (about 220 degrees Celsius) and let it preheat for about 20 minutes. Spray an 8-inch pizza pan with some cooking spray.

2. Combine the gluten free all-purpose flour, cornstarch, Parmesan cheese, xanthan gum, oregano, garbanzo bean flour, tapioca starch, baking powder, Italian seasoning and salt together in a large mixing bowl. Keep it aside.

3. Place the sugar in a small mixing bowl and add in some lukewarm water. Mix well until the sugar is dissolved. Sprinkle the active dry yeast over the sugar water and keep t aside for 4 to 5 minutes or until the yeast is foamy.

4. In another large mixing bowl combine the egg, olive oil, white sugar, vinegar and garlic together. Whisk well until all the *ingredients* are well combined.

5. Add the prepared yeast mixture to the egg mixture and whisk well.

6.   Add the flour mix to the egg and yeast mix and mix well to form a smooth and lump free dough.

7.   Transfer the dough to the greased pizza pan and gently spread it, keeping the center thin and edges slightly thicker.

8.   Pop the pizza pan into the preheated oven and bake for about 12 to 15 minutes or until the dough rises.

9.   Top the pizza crust with your favorite gluten free toppings and continue baking for another 25 to 30 minutes or until the crust is a delicious golden brown.

10.   If you want a crispier crust, remove the prepared pizza from the pizza pan and place it directly on the rack in the oven. Cook for another 5 minutes.

11.   Serve hot.

12.   Enjoy!

Quinoa Stuffed Pork Tenderloin

Serves: 2

Ingredients

- 2 tablespoons uncooked quinoa
- 1 tablespoon olive oil
- 1/4 cup water
- 1/4 onion, chopped
- 1/2 small apple, peel and core removed, chopped
- 1 clove garlic, chopped
- 2 tablespoons raisins
- 2 mushrooms, chopped
- Freshly ground black pepper, to taste
- 1 tablespoon pine nuts
- 1 tablespoon white wine
- 1/2 pinch ground cinnamon
- 1 pork tenderloin (1/2 pound)
- Garam masala as per taste (can be found at your nearest Indian or Pakistani store)
- Salt, to taste

Directions

1. Place the quinoa in a saucepan and pour the water over it. Heat the saucepan over a medium high flame and heat until the mixture is boiling.

2. Reduce the heat to a medium low and cover the saucepan with a lid. Continue simmering the quinoa on a medium low flame for about 15 to 17 minutes or until the quinoa has absorbed all the water and has become tender.

3. Pour the olive oil into a skillet and heat over a medium low flame. Add the onion, apples, pine nuts, garlic, raisins, and mushrooms to the pan. Cook and stir constantly, until the onion turns translucent and becomes tender.

4. Add the white wine to the pan and cook for another minute or two until the wine completely evaporates.

5. Add the contents of the pan to the cooked quinoa and mix well. Set aside.

6. Crank up your oven to 425 degrees Fahrenheit (220 degrees Celsius) and let the oven preheat for about 20 minutes.

7. Carefully slice open the pork tenderloin horizontally from the middle until you are about half an inch away from the other end. Open the pork flat, like a book.

8. Cover a flat and solid surface using a plastic wrap and place the open pork tenderloin on it. Cover with another sheet of plastic wrap. Use the smooth side of a mallet or the bottom of a flat saucepan to firmly pound on the tenderloin until it is about half an inch thick.

9. Sprinkle both sides of the flattened tenderloin with cinnamon, salt, garam masala and black pepper. Carefully spoon the prepared apple and quinoa filling on the pork tenderloin.

10. Carefully roll the pork tenderloin tightly and secure the roll in place using toothpicks or a twine.

11. Place the pork roll in a roasting pan and pop the pan into the preheated oven. Bake for about 35 to 40 minutes or until a thermometer inserted in the center of the roll reads 145 degrees Fahrenheit (63 degrees Celsius) and the pork is no longer pink in the center.

12. Cover the pan with an aluminum foil and let the roll rest for about 10 to 15 minutes before slicing.

13. Slice and serve hot with a gluten free condiment of your choice.

14. Enjoy!

Caramel Apple Pork Chops

Serves: 2

Ingredients

- 2 (3/4 inch) thick pork chops
- 1 tablespoon brown sugar
- 1/2 teaspoon vegetable oil
- Salt, to taste
- 1/8 teaspoon ground cinnamon
- Freshly ground black pepper, to taste
- 1/8 teaspoon ground nutmeg
- 1 tart apple – peel and core removed, sliced thinly
- 1 tablespoon unsalted butter
- 4 1/2 teaspoons pecans (optional)

Directions

1. Crank up your oven to 175 degrees Fahrenheit (about 80 degrees Celsius) and let it preheat for about 20 minutes. Place a medium sized dish in the oven so that it can become warm.
2. Place a large sized skillet over a medium high flame and spray with some cooking oil. Once the pan is smoking, lightly brush the pork chops with some oil and place them in the smoking pan.
3. Cook the pork chops for about 5 to 7 minutes, flipping them around every minute or so or until the pork chops are cooked through.
4. Transfer the pan-fried pork chops to the warm baking dish and keep it in the oven so that the pork chops stay warm.
5. Combine the brown sugar, black pepper, nutmeg, salt and cinnamon together in a small mixing bowl.
6. Place the butter in the skillet and heat over a medium low flame until the butter melts. Add the seasoning mix and apple slices to the butter.
7. Cover the skillet with the lid and cook for about 5 to 7 minutes or until the apple slices are tender. Drain the apple slices and place them over the prepared pork chops. Return the dish back into the oven.
8. Continue cooking the sauce in the skillet until it thickens and coats the back of your spoon.
9. Gently pour the prepared sauce over the pork chops and apples.
10. Serve hot topped with some pecans if you like.
11. Enjoy!

Slow Cooked Pulled BBQ Pork

Serves: 6

Ingredients

- 1/2 (14 ounce) can beef broth
- 1/2 (18 ounce) bottle barbeque sauce
- 1 and a 1/2 pounds boneless pork ribs

Directions

1. Place the boneless pork ribs in the bottom of a slow cooker.

2. Gently pour the beef broth over the pork ribs.

3. Cover and cook on the High setting for about 4 hours or until the meat is extremely tender and can be shredded easily.

4. Remove the pork ribs from the slow cooker and place in a flat dish.

5. Once cool enough to handle, use two forks to gently shred the pork ribs.

6. Crank up your oven to 350 degrees Fahrenheit (about 175 degrees Celsius) and let it preheat for about 20 minutes.

7. Place the shredded pork ribs in a cast iron skillet or in a Dutch oven and add the barbeque sauce to it.

8. Mix well and pop the baking dish into the preheated oven and bake for about 30 to 35 minutes or until the pork is thoroughly heated.

9. Serve hot in a gluten free bun.

10. Enjoy!

Cabbage Roll Casserole

Serves: 6

Ingredients

- 1 pound ground beef
- 1/2 (29 ounce) can tomato sauce
- 1/2 cup chopped onion
- 1 and 3/4 pounds chopped cabbage
- 1/2 teaspoon salt
- 1/2 cup uncooked white rice
- 1 (14 ounce) can beef broth

Directions

1. Crank up your oven to 350 degrees Fahrenheit (about 175 degrees Celsius) and let it preheat for about 20 minutes.

2. Add some oil to a large skillet and heat over a medium high flame until smoking. Add in the beef and cook until the beef is well browned and has lost all its redness. Drain all the extra fat from it.

3. Combine the onion, cabbage, salt, tomato sauce, and rice together in a large mixing bowl. Mix well until well combined.

4. Add in the browned beef and pour the prepared mixture into a 9 inches by 13 inches baking dish.

5. Pour the beef broth over the meat mixture and cover the baking dish with some heavy-duty aluminum foil.

6. Pop the covered baking dish into the preheated oven and bake for about an hour.

7. Remove the baking dish from the oven and remove the foil from the baking dish and give the contents of the baking dish a stir.

8. Replace the cover and bake for an additional 25 to 35 minutes.

9. Remove the baking dish from the oven and rest the dish, covered, for about 10 minutes.

10. Serve hot.

11. Enjoy!

Infallible Rib Roast

Serves: 3

Ingredients

- 1 (2.5 pound) standing beef rib roast
- 1/2 teaspoon ground black pepper
- 1 teaspoon salt
- 1/2 teaspoon garlic powder

Directions

1. Remove the roast from the refrigerator and set aside for at least one hour or until it reaches room temperature.

2. Crank up your oven to 375 degrees Fahrenheit (about 190 degrees Celsius) and let it preheat for at least 20 minutes.

3. In a small mixing bowl combine the salt, garlic powder and pepper together.

4. Place the roast in a roasting pan with its rib side down and fatty side up. Pour the seasoning mix over the roast and rub it in using your fingers.

5. Pop the roasting pan into the oven and roast the beef rib roast for an hour. When the hour is up, turn off the oven and leave the roasting pan inside for about 3 to 4 hours. Do not open the oven door.

6. About an hour before serving, turn the oven on again at 375 degrees Fahrenheit (about 190 degrees Celsius) and re-heat the roast until the internal temperature of the roast reaches 145 degrees Fahrenheit (about 62 degrees Celsius).

7. Remove the roast from the oven and rest it for about 10 to 12 minutes before slicing.

8. Serve hot.

9. Enjoy!

Beef and Rice Stuffed Peppers

Serves: 3

Ingredients
- 1/2 pound ground beef
- 1/2 cup water
- 1/4 cup uncooked long grain white rice
- 3 green bell peppers
- 1 and a 1/2 teaspoons Worcestershire sauce
- 1 (8 ounce) can tomato sauce
- 1/8 teaspoon garlic powder
- Salt, to taste
- 1/8 teaspoon onion powder
- 1/2 teaspoon Italian seasoning
- Freshly ground black pepper, to taste

Directions

1. Crank up your oven to 350 degrees Fahrenheit (about 175 degrees Celsius) and let it preheat for about 20 minutes.
2. Pour the water into a saucepan and add the uncooked white rice to it. Heat the saucepan over a high flame until the water is boiling. Reduce the heat to a medium low and cook the rice for about 20 minutes.
3. Add the beef to a thick-bottomed skillet and cook over a medium high flame until the beef is well browned and loses all its redness.
4. Carefully slice the tops of the bell peppers. Using a spoon, remove the membranes and the seeds from inside the bell peppers. If the bell peppers have uneven bottoms, slice the bell peppers slightly so that you have an even base.
5. Place the bell peppers in a baking dish with the hollowed end pointed upward.
6. Combine the cooked rice, Worcestershire sauce, onion powder, pepper, browned beef, ½ can tomato sauce, garlic powder and salt together in a large mixing bowl. Mix well until well combined.
7. Divide the prepared mix in three equal parts and spoon it into the bell pepper hollows.
8. In another mixing bowl, combine the remaining tomato sauce and Italian seasoning together. Mix well until well incorporated.
9. Spoon the prepared sauce over the rice and beef mix in the bell peppers.
10. Pop the baking dish into the preheated oven and bake for about an hour, basting the outsides of the bell peppers with the sauce every 15 minutes to keep them moist.
11. Serve hot.
12. Enjoy!

Blackened Chicken

Serves: 1

Ingredients

- 1 skinless, boneless chicken breast half
- 1/4 teaspoon paprika
- 1/8 teaspoon cayenne pepper
- 1/8 teaspoon salt
- 1/8 teaspoon ground cumin
- 1/8 teaspoon ground white pepper
- 1/8 teaspoon dried thyme
- 1/8 teaspoon onion powder

Directions

1. Crank up your oven to 350 degrees Fahrenheit (about 175 degrees Celsius) and let it preheat for about 20 minutes. Lightly spray a baking sheet with some cooking spray.

2. Place a cast iron skillet on the stove and heat on a high flame for about 5 to 7 minutes or until it is smoking hot.

3. Combine the paprika, cayenne, thyme, onion powder, salt, cumin and white pepper together in a small mixing bowl.

4. Apply some oil all over the chicken breast or spray it with some cooking spray on both sides.

5. Sprinkle the spice mixture all over the oiled chicken breast on both the sides and rub the spice mixture in using your fingers.

6. Place the oil and spice coated chicken breast on the hot skillet and cook for about 1 minute.

7. Flip it over and continue cooking the other side for another minute.

8. Remove the chicken breast from the skillet and place on the prepared baking sheet.

9. Pop the baking sheet into the preheated oven and bake for about 5 to 7 minutes or until the juices run clear and the center of the chicken breast is no longer pink.

10. Serve hot, topped with your favorite gluten free sauce and with some grilled or steamed vegetables on the side.

11. Enjoy!

Lamb Chops with Balsamic Reduction

Serves: 2

Ingredients
- 1/2 teaspoon dried rosemary
- 1/4 teaspoon dried thyme
- 1/8 teaspoon dried basil
- Salt, to taste
- 2 lamb chops (3/4 inch thick)
- Freshly ground black pepper, to taste
- 1 and a 1/2 teaspoons olive oil
- 8 teaspoons aged balsamic vinegar
- 2 tablespoons minced shallots
- 1 and a 1/2 teaspoons butter
- 6 tablespoons chicken broth

Directions

1. Combine the rosemary, thyme, pepper, basil and salt together in a cup or a small mixing bowl.
2. Sprinkle this mixture on the lamb chops and rub it on both sides of the chop.
3. Place the lamb chops in a plate and cover. Keep aside for about 15 to 20 minutes so that they can absorb the flavors of the spice rub.
4. Pour the olive oil into a large skillet and heat over a medium high flame until the oil is lightly smoking.
5. Placc the spice rub covered lamb chops in the skillet and cook them for about 4 minutes per side for a medium rare cook or continue cooking for a longer time until the lamb achieves the desired degree of doneness.
6. Remove the lamb chops from the skillets and set aside.
7. Place the shallots in the skillet and cook for 4 to 5 minutes or until the shallots are well browned.
8. Add the vinegar to the pan and gently scrub the pan with your spoon so that the browned bits that are stuck to the pan come unstuck.
9. Pour in the chicken broth and continue cooking on a medium high flame, while stirring it occasionally. Cook the sauce for about 5 to 7 minutes or until the sauce is reduced to half of what it originally was.
10. Take the skillet off the heat and add the butter to the sauce and mix well until well incorporated.
11. Pour the prepared cause over the lamb chops.
12. Serve immediately with a side of mashed potatoes.
13. Enjoy!

Slow Cooked Hot Mexican Style Meat

Serves: 6

Ingredients

- 1 (2 pound) chuck roast
- 1/2 teaspoon ground black pepper
- 1/2 teaspoon salt
- 1 tablespoon olive oil
- 10 tablespoons diced green chili pepper
- 1/2 large onion, chopped
- 1/2 teaspoon chili powder
- 1/2 (5 ounce) bottle hot pepper sauce
- 1/2 teaspoon ground cayenne pepper
- 1/2 teaspoon garlic powder

Directions

1. Trim all the extra fat from the chuck roast and sprinkle salt and pepper over it. Use your fingers to lightly rub the salt and pepper into the roast.
2. Pour the olive oil into a large skillet and heat over a medium high flame until it is lightly smoking.
3. Add the chuck roast to the skillet and cook until well browned on all sides.
4. Transfer the browned beef to the bottom of a slow cooker and top it with the chopped onion.
5. Add in the green chili pepper, cayenne pepper, garlic powder, chili powder and hot pepper sauce over the chuck roast.
6. Pour in enough water so that about 1/3rd of the roast is covered.
7. Cover the Slow Cooker, and cook on the High setting for about 6 hours, checking every hour if there is enough cooking liquid in the slow cooker. If all the liquid is gone, add in a little at a time to keep the chuck roast moist and juicy.
8. At the end of 6 hours, lower the heat setting and continue cooking for another 3 to 4 hours or until the roast is tender enough to fall apart.
9. Transfer the meat to a bowl and shred using two forks.
10. Pour the cooking liquid into a skillet and heat until bubbling. Reduce the heat to a low flame and continue simmering the liquid until it thickens and is thick enough to coat the back of the spoon.
11. Add the shredded meat to the sauce and mix well.
12. Spoon into some gluten free tacos or gluten free tortillas and serve hot.
13. Enjoy!

Spicy and Tangy Chicken Kabobs

Serves: 2

Ingredients

- 1/2 pound chicken breast halves, skinless and boneless - cut into 1 1/2 inch pieces
- 4 and 1/2 teaspoons olive oil
- 1/2 lime, juiced
- 2 and 1/4 teaspoons red wine vinegar
- 1/2 teaspoon chili powder
- 1/4 teaspoon onion powder
- 1/4 teaspoon paprika
- 1/4 teaspoon garlic powder
- Salt, to taste
- Cayenne pepper, to taste
- Freshly ground black pepper, to taste

Directions

1. Pour the olive oil into a small mixing bowl. Add in the lime juice and vinegar and whisk well until all the liquids are well emulsified.

2. Add in the chili powder, onion powder, cayenne pepper, black pepper, paprika, garlic powder and salt. Mix well.

3. Place the chicken breasts pieces in a shallow baking dish. Pour the prepared spiced oil over them and toss well until well coated.

4. Cover the baking dish using a plastic wrap and refrigerate for at least 2 hours.

5. Turn on your grill on the medium high setting and preheat for about 10 to 12 minutes.

6. Drain the chicken pieces from the marinade and thread them onto the skewers. Keep the size of your grill in mind so that you don't end up threading too many pieces on a single skewer. If using wooden or bamboo skewers, soak them for about half an hour in warm water before using. Discard the leftover marinade.

7. Brush some oil on the grate and place the skewers on the hot grill. Cook for about 7 to 8 minutes per side or until the juices run clear.

8. Serve hot with your favorite gluten free condiment.

9. Enjoy!

Cornish Game Hens with Garlic and Rosemary

Serves: 2

Ingredients

- 2 Cornish game hens
- Freshly ground black pepper, to taste
- Salt, to taste
- 1/2 lemon, quartered
- 4 1/2 teaspoons olive oil
- 2 sprigs fresh rosemary
- 12 cloves garlic
- 8 teaspoons chicken broth, low sodium
- 8 teaspoons white wine
- 2 sprigs fresh rosemary, for garnish

Directions

1. Crank up your oven to 450 degrees F (230 degrees C) and let it preheat for about 20 minutes.

2. Rub about 1 tablespoon of olive oil over each Cornish hen and lightly sprinkle some salt and pepper over them.

3. Place 1 rosemary sprig and 1 lemon wedge in the cavity of each hen.

4. Place the hens in a large roasting pan and place the garlic cloves around the hens.

5. Pop the roasting pan into the preheated oven and roast for about 20 to 25 minutes. Reduce the temperature of the oven to about 350 degrees Fahrenheit (175 degrees Celsius).

6. Combine the wine, remaining oil and chicken broth together in a large mixing bowl. Whisk well until well combined.

7. Pour the prepared oil mix over the hens and continue roasting in the oven for about 20 to 25 minutes more or until the juices run clear and the hens have a golden brown exterior. Make sure you baste the hens with the juices from the pan at 10-minute intervals to keep them juicy and moist.

8. Carefully extract the hens from the pan, emptying all the juices from the cavity into the pan, and place them on a platter. Make a tent using an aluminum foil and cover the hens.

9. Pour the juices from the pan, along with the garlic cloves, into a medium sized saucepan and heat over a high flame until boiling.

10. Reduce the heat to a medium low and continue heating the sauce until it reduces and has a sauce like consistency.

11. Cut the hens into two halves lengthwise and place on a platter. Spoon the prepared sauce over the hen halves and garnish with rosemary sprigs.

12. Serve hot.

13. Enjoy!

Delicious Dill Chickpea Sandwich Filling

Serves: 6

Ingredients

- 2 (19 ounce) cans garbanzo beans,
- 1 onion, chopped
- 2 stalks celery, chopped
- 2 tablespoons mayonnaise
- 2 teaspoons dried dill weed
- 2 tablespoons lemon juice
- Freshly ground black pepper, to taste
- Salt, to taste

Directions

1. Drain the garbanzo beans from the canning liquid and rinse well. Spread on a kitchen towel and pat dry.

2. Transfer the chickpeas into a medium sized mixing bowl and mash using a masher or the back of a spoon until they get a paste like consistency.

3. Add the celery, mayonnaise, dill, pepper, onion, lemon juice and salt to the mashed garbanzo beans and mix well until all the *ingredients* are well incorporated.

4. Spread over some toasted gluten free bread and serve immediately.

5. Enjoy!

Garlic Butter Sirloin Steak

Serves: 4

Ingredients

- 2 pounds beef sirloin steaks
- 1/4 cup butter
- 1 teaspoon garlic powder
- 2 cloves garlic, minced
- Freshly ground black pepper, to taste
- Salt, to taste

Directions

1. Turn up your grill to the high heat setting and let it preheat.

2. Place the butter in a small saucepan and heat over a medium low flame until melted.

3. Add the minced garlic and garlic powder to the melted butter and mix well. Keep aside.

4. Sprinkle both sides of the steak with generous amounts of salt and pepper. Rub in the seasonings using your fingers.

5. Place the seasoned steaks on the hot grill and grill for about 4 to 6 minutes on each side for medium rare doneness. Cooking time will vary according to the doneness desired.

6. When the steaks are done to your desired doneness, transfer to warm serving plates.

7. Lightly spoon the prepared sauce over the steaks and let the steaks rest for about 4 minutes before serving.

8. Serve hot with a side of mashed potatoes.

9. Enjoy!

Slow Cooked Barbeque Chuck Roast

Serves: 4

Ingredients

- 1 (1.5 pound) boneless chuck roast
- 1/2 teaspoon onion powder
- 1/2 teaspoon garlic powder
- Salt, to taste
- 1/2 (18 ounce) bottle barbeque sauce
- Freshly ground black pepper, to taste

Directions

1. Place the roast in the bottom of a slow cooker.

2. Combine the onion powder, salt, pepper and garlic powder together in a small mixing bowl.

3. Sprinkle the prepared seasoning mix all over the chuck roast, rubbing the seasoning into the meat.

4. Pour the barbeque sauce over the seasoned meat.

5. Cover the slow cooker and cook the Low setting for about 6 to 8 hours.

6. Once done, extract the meat from the slow cooker and shred using two forks.

7. Transfer the shredded meat back into the slow cooker.

8. Cover with a lid and continue cooking on the Low setting for another hour or so.

9. Serve hot.

10. Enjoy!

Chapter 8: Bread & Side Recipes

Fluffy Gluten Free Cornbread

Serves: 6

Ingredients

- 1 egg, lightly beaten
- 2 tablespoons vegetable oil
- 3/4 cup lukewarm water
- 3/4 cup fine cornmeal
- 1/2 cup rice flour
- 1/2 cup millet flour
- 2 tablespoons white sugar
- 1/2 teaspoon salt
- 1 ½ teaspoons baking powder

Directions

1. Crank up your oven to 400 degrees F (200 degrees C) and let it preheat for about 20 minutes. Lightly grease a 7 inches by 7 inches baking pan with some oil.

2. Add the egg, vegetable oil and water together in a bowl and whisk until all the liquids are well emulsified.

3. Combine the cornmeal, rice flour, baking powder, millet flour, sugar and salt together in another large mixing bowl.

4. Use your fingers to make a small well in the center of the *ingredients*.

5. Pour the wet *ingredients* into the well and lightly mix using until the *ingredients* are well combined.

6. Pour the prepared batter into the greased baking dish and lightly pat it on the counter to get rid of air bubbles.

7. Pop the baking dish into the preheated oven and bake for about 20 to 25 minutes or until the bread springs back when lightly pressed and has a golden exterior.

8. Cool the bread in pan for about 10 minutes before removing it from the pan.

9. Cool the bread on a wire rack for another 15 minutes.

10. Slice and serve.

11. Enjoy!

Gluten Free Banana Bread

Serves: 8

Ingredients

- 1 cup gluten free all-purpose baking flour
- 1/4 teaspoon salt
- 1/2 teaspoon baking powder
- 1/4 cup butter
- 1 egg, lightly beaten
- 1/4 cup turbinado sugar
- 3 ripe bananas, mashed
- 4 ½ teaspoons maple syrup

Directions

1. Crank up your oven to 350 degrees Fahrenheit (175 degrees Celsius) and let it preheat for about 20 minutes. Lightly grease a 9 inches by 5 inches loaf pan with some oil.

2. Combine the gluten free all-purpose flour, salt and baking power together in a large mixing bowl.

3. Add the sugar and butter to another bowl and cream using and electronic blender. Add in the egg, mashed bananas and maple syrup to the creamed butter and continue blending until all the *ingredients* are well combined.

4. Add the banana mix to the bowl with the flour mix and mix well until all the *ingredients* are well incorporated.

5. Pour the prepared batter into the loaf pan.

6. Pop the loaf pan into the preheated oven and bake for about 25 to 35 minutes.

7. Cool the bread in the loaf pan for about 10 minutes before cooling completely on a wire rack.

8. Slice and serve.

9. Enjoy!

10. (If you do not have a loaf pan, you can make this bread in muffin tins. Bake the muffin tins for about 15 minutes or until a toothpick inserted in the center of the tin comes out clean.)

Gluten Free Zucchini Bread

Serves: 5

Ingredients

- 1/2 cup diced zucchini
- 1/4 cup canola oil
- 1 egg
- 1/2 teaspoon gluten free vanilla extract
- 1/4 cup white rice flour
- 1/2 cup white sugar
- 1/4 cup sweet rice flour
- 1 tablespoon tapioca starch
- 1/4 cup cornstarch
- 1/2 teaspoon baking powder
- 1/4 teaspoon baking soda
- 1/4 teaspoon salt
- 1/2 teaspoon ground cinnamon
- 1/4 teaspoon xanthan gum

For the Glaze:

- 1/2 teaspoon lemon juice
- 1 ½ teaspoons confectioners' sugar

Directions

1. Crank up your oven to 325 degrees Fahrenheit (165 degrees Celsius) and let it preheat for about 20 minutes. Lightly grease a 9 inches by 5 inches loaf pan with some oil.

2. Place the zucchini, oil, egg and vanilla extract together in the jar of a blender. Blitz until all the *ingredients* are well combined and the mix has the texture of a thick milkshake.

3. Combine the white sugar, sweet rice flour, tapioca cinnamon, xanthan gum, white rice flour, cornstarch, baking powder, baking soda and salt together in a large mixing bowl. Whisk until well combined.

4. Pour the contents of the blender into the bowl with the dry *ingredients* and mix well to form a smooth and lump free batter.

5. Pour the batter into the loaf pan.

6. Pop the loaf pan into the preheated oven and bake for about an hour.

7. Cool the bread in the loaf pan for about 10 minutes before cooling completely on a wire rack.

8. Combine the lemon juice and confectioner's sugar in small bowl and pour it over the loaf.

9. Serve immediately.

10. Enjoy!

Gluten Free Bread Machine White Bread

Serves: 6

Ingredients

- 1 ½ eggs
- 2 tablespoons olive oil
- 1 ½ teaspoons cider vinegar
- 2 tablespoons honey
- 1/2 teaspoon salt
- 3/4 cup buttermilk, at room temperature
- 1 ½ teaspoons xanthan gum
- 1/4 cup potato starch
- 2 tablespoons and 2 teaspoons cornstarch
- 1/4 cup soy flour
- 1 ½ teaspoons active dry yeast
- 1 cup white rice flour

Directions

1. Follow the instructions of the manufacturer and place the *ingredients* in the bread machine as recommended by the manufacturer.

2. Run the bread machine on the sweet dough cycle and not the gluten free cycle.

3. 5 minutes after starting the cycle, check the consistency of the dough. Add more liquid or flour if necessary.

4. When the cycle is completed, let the bread cool in the pan for about 15 to 20 minutes.

5. Cool on a wire rack.

6. Slice and serve.

7. Enjoy!

Gluten Free Irish Soda Bread

Serves: 4

Ingredients

- 1/2 cup buttermilk
- 3/4 cup white rice flour
- 1/4 cup white sugar
- 1/4 cup tapioca flour
- 1/2 teaspoon baking soda
- 1/2 teaspoon salt
- 1/2 teaspoon baking powder
- 1/2 egg

Directions

1. Crank up your oven to 350 degrees Fahrenheit (175 degrees Celsius) and let it preheat for about 20 minutes. Lightly grease a 9-inch round cake pan with some oil.

2. In a large mixing bowl, add together the rice flour, sugar, baking powder, tapioca flour, baking soda and salt, mix well until well combined. Make a shallow well in the center of the dry *ingredients* using your fingers.

3. Add the buttermilk and egg together in another mixing bowl. Whisk well until well combined.

4. Pour the wet *ingredients* into the well in the dry *ingredients*. Mix well until the dry *ingredients* are well moistened.

5. Pour the prepared batter into the greased cake tin.

6. Pop the cake tin into the preheated oven and bake for about 60 to 70 minutes or until a knife inserted in the center of the tin comes out clean.

7. Cool the bread in the pan for about 10 to 15 minutes before removing from the pan. Cool on a wire rack for another 15 to 20 minutes or until completely cool.

8. Wrap the bread in some aluminum foil or plastic wrap and set the bread aside for a few hours to get the best flavor.

9. Slice and serve.

10. Enjoy!

Pao de Queijo – The Brazilian Cheese Bread

Serves: 3

Ingredients

- ¼ cup olive oil or butter
- 8 teaspoons soy milk or milk
- 8 teaspoons water
- ½ teaspoon salt
- 1 teaspoon minced garlic
- 1 cup tapioca flour
- 1 beaten egg
- 1/3 cup freshly grated Parmesan cheese

Directions

1. Crank up your oven to 375 degrees Fahrenheit (about 190 degrees Celsius) and let it preheat for about 20 minutes.

2. Pour the olive oil (or butter), salt and milk (or soy milk) into a large saucepan. Heat over a high flame until the mixture is lightly bubbling.

3. Take the pan off heat and immediately add the garlic and tapioca flour to it. Mix well until it forms a smooth and lump free mixture. Keep aside for 15 to 20 minutes.

4. Add the egg and cheese into the saucepan with the tapioca mixture and mix vigorously until all the *ingredients* are well incorporated. The mixture will have the consistency of cottage cheese.

5. Scoop out about ¼ cup of the batter and shape it into a small ball.

6. Place the mixture balls on an ungreased and unlined baking sheet.

7. Pop the baking sheet into the preheated oven and bake for about 20 to 25 minutes or until the bread gets a crispy golden brown exterior.

8. Serve warm.

9. Enjoy!

Light and Fluffy Cloud Bread

Serves: 10

Ingredients

- 6 large eggs, separated
- 1/4 pound cream cheese, very soft
- 1/2 teaspoon cream of tartar
- 2 tablespoons white sugar

Directions

1. Crank up your oven to 350 degrees Fahrenheit (about 175 degrees Celsius) and let it preheat for about 20 minutes. Lightly rub some oil on a baking sheet and place a parchment sheet over it.

2. Place the egg whites in a large bowl. Add in the cream of tartar and beat until there are stiff peaks.

3. In another mixing bowl, combine the egg yolks, sugar and cream cheese together using a flat wooden spoon. Once the *ingredients* are roughly combined, blend the mixture together using an electric beater until the cream cheese is completely incorporated.

4. Slowly add the egg whites to the egg yolk and cream cheese mixture. Use an extremely light hand while mixing to ensure that the egg whites do not end up deflating.

5. Scoop out the mixture and make 5 to 6 rough "buns" on the parchment lined baking sheet.

6. Pop the baking sheet into the preheated oven and bake for about 30 minutes or until the bread has a light golden brown exterior.

7. Serve warm with some eggs.

8. Enjoy!

Roasted Brussels sprouts

Serves: 3

Ingredients

- 3/4 pound Brussels sprouts, yellow leaves removed and ends trimmed
- 1/2 teaspoon kosher salt
- 4 1/2 teaspoons olive oil
- 1/4 teaspoon freshly ground black pepper

Directions

1. Crank up your oven to 400 degrees Fahrenheit (about 205 degrees Celsius) and let it preheat for about 20 minutes.

2. In a large mixing bowl add the Brussels sprouts, kosher salt, olive oil and pepper and mix well until the Brussels sprouts are well coated. You can even use a re-sealable bag to toss the Brussels sprouts with the oil and seasonings.

3. Transfer the oil and seasoning coated Brussels sprouts onto an ungreased baking sheet.

4. Pop the baking sheet into the preheated oven and place it on the center rack.

5. Roast the Brussels sprouts for about 35 to 50 minutes, pausing the oven every 6 to 8 minutes in order to toss the Brussels sprouts around to ensure even browning. Reduce the heat if the Brussels sprouts are burning.

6. When the Brussels sprouts turn a really dark brown, almost close to black, the Brussels sprouts are done. Taste and adjust seasoning.

7. Serve immediately.

8. Enjoy!

Grilled Asparagus Spears

Serves: 2

Ingredients

- ½ pound fresh asparagus spears, trimmed
- Salt, to taste
- 1 1/2 teaspoons olive oil
- Freshly ground black pepper, to taste

Directions

1. Turn on your grill on the high heat setting and let the grill heat up for about 10 to 15 minutes.

2. Place the asparagus spears in a large bowl.

3. Pour in the oil and toss until the asparagus is well coated by the oil.

4. Season to taste with salt and pepper.

5. Place the asparagus spears on the hot grill and grill for about 3 to 4 minutes, or until they reach the desired level of doneness.

6. Serve immediately.

7. Enjoy!

Green Beans with Cherry Tomatoes

Serves: 3

Ingredients

- ¾ pound green beans, ends trimmed and chopped into 2 inch pieces
- 1 cup cherry tomato halves
- 2 tablespoons butter
- ¾ cup water
- 1 ½ teaspoons sugar
- 1/8 teaspoon pepper
- 1/4 teaspoon garlic salt
- 3/4 teaspoon chopped fresh basil

Directions

1. Pour the water into a large saucepan. Add the green bean pieces, cover with a lid and heat he saucepan over a high flame until the water is boiling. Lower the heat to low and let the water simmer for about 10 to 12 minutes. Drain the water and keep the green beans aside.

2. Place the butter in a skillet and heat over a medium low flame. Once the butter has melted, add in the sugar, salt, basil, garlic and pepper and mix well.

3. Add the tomatoes to the herbed butter and mix well. Cook until slightly tender.

4. Arrange the green beans in a serving plate and pour the tomato mixture over them. Toss gently until well coated.

5. Serve immediately.

6. Enjoy!

Spicy Quinoa with Corn and Black Beans

Serves: 5

Ingredients

- ½ teaspoon vegetable oil
- 1 ½ cloves garlic, chopped
- 1/2 onion, chopped
- 6 tablespoons quinoa
- 1/2 teaspoon ground cumin
- 3/4 cup vegetable broth
- 1/8 teaspoon cayenne pepper
- Freshly ground black pepper, to taste
- Salt, to taste
- 1/2 cup frozen corn kernels
- 1/4 cup chopped fresh cilantro
- 1 (15 ounce) can black beans, drained and rinsed

Directions

1. Pour the oil into a saucepan and heat over a medium flame. Once the oil is hot enough, add in the garlic and onion to the saucepan and cook for about 8 to 10 minutes or until they are well browned.

2. Add the quinoa to the sautéed onion and garlic. Mix well.

3. Pour in the vegetable broth and add cumin, salt, cayenne pepper and pepper to the saucepan.

4. Heat on a high flame until the mixture is boiling.

5. Cover the saucepan with a lid and reduce the flame to a low. Cook for about 20 to 25 minutes or until the quinoa has absorbed all the water and has softened.

6. Add the frozen corn to the quinoa and mix well. Continue cooking for about 5 minutes until the corn is well heated through.

7. Add in the black beans and cilantro. Mix well.

8. Serve hot.

9. Enjoy!

Tangy Harvest Rice Dish

Serves: 3

Ingredients

- 1/4 cup slivered almonds
- 1/4 cup uncooked brown rice
- 1 cup chicken broth
- 1/4 cup uncooked wild rice
- 1 ½ onions, sliced into 1/2 inch wedges
- 4 ½ teaspoons butter
- 1 ½ teaspoons brown sugar
- 1/3 cup fresh sliced mushrooms
- ½ cup dried cranberries
- ¼ teaspoon orange zest
- Freshly ground black pepper, to taste
- Salt, to taste

Directions

1. Spread the almonds in a single layer in an ungreased baking dish. Pop the baking dish into the oven and turn it up to 350 degrees Fahrenheit (175 degrees Celsius). Toast the almonds for about 8 to 10 minutes or until well browned.

2. Combine the broth, wild rice and brown rice together in a medium sized saucepan. Heat over a high flame until the mixture is boiling.

3. Reduce the heat to a low flame and cover the saucepan with a lid. Let the mix simmer for about 45 to 50 minutes or until all the broth is absorbed and the rice is tender.

4. While the rice cooks, heat the butter on a medium high flame in a medium sized skillet. Add the brown sugar and onions to the butter and cook until all the butter is absorbed and the onions are tender and translucent. Reduce the flame to low and continue cooking the onions for an additional 20 minutes or until the onions are well browned and caramelized.

5. Add the mushrooms and cranberries to the skillet. Cover the skillet and cook for about 10 to 12 minutes or until the berries are swollen. Add the orange zest and almonds to the pan and mix well.

6. Pour the contents of the skillet onto the cooked rice. Season with salt and pepper.

7. Serve hot.

8. Enjoy!

Buttery Green Beans with Garlic

Serves: 10

Ingredients

- 2 tablespoons butter
- 2 medium heads garlic – peel removed and thinly sliced
- 8 tablespoons olive oil
- 4 (14.5 ounce) cans green beans, drained
- Freshly ground black pepper, to taste
- Salt, to taste
- ½ cup grated Parmesan cheese

Directions

1. Place the butter and olive oil together in a large skillet. Heat over a medium high flame until the butter melts.

2. Add the garlic to the pan and cook until the garlic is well browned. Stir constantly to ensure that it doesn't burn.

3. Add the green beans to the pan and season to taste with salt and pepper.

4. Cook for about 10 to 12 minutes or until the beans are tender.

5. Transfer the beans to serving plate.

6. Serve immediately topped with the Parmesan cheese.

7. Enjoy!

Boston Baked Beans

Serves: 3

Ingredients

- 1 cup navy beans
- ½ onion, finely diced
- ¼ pound bacon
- 4 ½ teaspoons molasses
- 1/8 teaspoon ground black pepper
- 1 teaspoon salt
- 1/8 teaspoon dry mustard
- 1 ½ teaspoons Worcestershire sauce
- 1/4 cup ketchup
- 2 tablespoons brown sugar

Directions

1. Place the navy beans in a large bowl. Cover with cold water and leave overnight to soak.
2. Pour the beans and the soaking liquid into a saucepan. Heat over a high flame until bubbling. Lower the flame to a medium low and continue heating the beans for an hour or two, until the beans are softened but not mushy. Drain the beans and reserve the cooking liquid.
3. Crank up your oven to 325 degrees Fahrenheit (about 165 degrees Celsius) and let it preheat for about 20 minutes.
4. Spread the beans in the bottom of a casserole dish or a bean pot. Cover the beans with a layer of onion, topped with a layer of bacon.
5. Combine together the molasses, pepper, ketchup, brown sugar, salt, dry mustard and Worcestershire sauce together in a saucepan. Heat over a high flame until all the *ingredients* are well combined and the sauce is bubbling.
6. Pour the sauces over the beans. Add in enough of the reserved cooking liquid to cover the beans.
7. Cover the dish with some heavy-duty aluminum foil or a lid.
8. Pop the dish into the preheated oven and bake for 3 to 4 hours or until the beans are tender.
9. Around the halfway mark remove the aluminum foil or lid and give the beans a stir. Add in more cooking liquid if required.
10. Serve hot.

Slow Cooked Creamed Corn

Serves: 6

Ingredients

- 5/8 (16 ounce) package frozen corn kernels
- 1/4 cup butter
- 1/2 (8 ounce) package cream cheese
- 1/4 cup milk
- Salt, to taste
- 1 ½ teaspoons white sugar
- Freshly ground black pepper, to taste

Directions

1. Combine the cream cheese, milk and butter together in the bottom of a slow cooker.

2. Add in the sugar and mix well until the sugar has dissolved.

3. Add in the corn kernels and season to taste with the salt and pepper.

4. Cover the slow cooker and cook on the Low setting for 6 to 8 hour or on the High setting for 2 to 4 hours.

5. Serve warm with some fried chicken or roasted beef.

6. Enjoy!

Oven Roasted Sugar Snap Peas

Serves: 2

Ingredients

- ¼ pound sugar snap peas
- 1 ½ teaspoons chopped shallots
- 1 ½ teaspoons olive oil
- Kosher salt to taste
- ½ teaspoon chopped fresh thyme

Directions

1. Crank up your oven to 450 degrees Fahrenheit (about 230 degrees Celsius) and allow it to preheat for about 20 minutes.

2. Toss the sugar snap peas with some olive oil and spread them in a single layer on a baking sheet.

3. Sprinkle the shallots, kosher salt and thyme over them

4. Pop the baking sheet into the preheated oven and bake for about 7 to 9 minutes or until the sugar snap peas are softened, but firm.

5. Cool and serve.

6. Enjoy!

Creamy Roasted Garlic Mashed Potatoes

Serves: 4

Ingredients

- 3 cloves garlic, peeled
- 2 tablespoons olive oil
- 3 ½ baking potatoes, peeled and cubed
- 1/4 cup milk
- 2 tablespoons grated Parmesan cheese
- 1 tablespoon butter
- ¼ teaspoon salt
- 1/8 teaspoon ground black pepper

Directions

1. Crank up your oven to 350 degrees Fahrenheit (about 175 degrees Celsius) and let it preheat for about 20 minutes.

2. Arrange the garlic cloves in a small and shallow baking dish. Pour the olive oil over the cloves and cover the dish with a lid or with some aluminum foil.

3. Pop the dish into the oven and bake for about 40 to 45 minutes or until the garlic cloves are golden brown.

4. Salt a large pot of water and heat it over a high flame until it is boiling. Add the potatoes to the water and cook until the potatoes are tender, but firm enough to hold their shape.

5. Drain the potatoes from the water and transfer them to a large mixing bowl.

6. Add the roasted garlic, Parmesan cheese, milk and butter to the bowl with the potatoes. Season to taste with salt and pepper.

7. Use an electric mixer to blend the *ingredients* until they get to the consistency you desire.

8. Serve hot as a side with some roasted beef or pork ribs.

9. Enjoy!

Pan Tossed White Wine and Italian Herbed Mushrooms

Serves: 3

Ingredients

- 1 ½ teaspoons olive oil
- 1/2 teaspoon Italian seasoning
- ¾ pound fresh mushrooms
- 2 tablespoons dry white wine
- Salt, to taste
- 1 clove garlic, minced
- 1 tablespoon chopped fresh chives
- Freshly ground black pepper, to taste

Directions

1. Pour the oil into a skillet and heat over a medium high flame. Once the oil is hot, add the mushrooms to the skillet. Add in the Italian seasoning and cook for about 10 minutes or until the mushrooms start to shrink in size, while stirring constantly.

2. Pour the wine into the skillet and mix well. Add in the garlic and continue cooking until most of the wine evaporates.

3. Season to taste with salt and pepper.

4. Add in the chives and cook for an additional minute.

5. Serve hot.

6. Enjoy!

Chapter 9: Dessert Recipes

Chocolate Dipped Coconut Bon-Bons

Serves: 8

Ingredients

- 2 tablespoons butter
- 1/2 pound confectioners' sugar
- 1/2 cup sweetened condensed milk
- 1 cup flaked coconut
- 1 tablespoon shortening
- 4 ½ (1 ounce) squares semisweet chocolate

Directions

1. Combine the butter, sweetened condensed milk and confectioner's sugar together in a medium sized mixing bowl. Mix well until well combined.

2. Add in the flaked coconut and mix well to form a dough.

3. Scoop out about 1 tablespoon of the mix and roll it into 1-inch balls.

4. Arrange the balls in a shallow dish and refrigerate for 2 to 3 hours.

5. Place the shortening with chocolate in a heat safe bowl and place it over a double boiler. Ensure that the bottom of the bowl does not touch the surface of the water.

6. When the chocolate is melted, take it off heat and mix well until the shortening is incorporated with the chocolate.

7. Pierce the prepared chocolate balls with a toothpick and dip them in the chocolate and shortening mixture.

8. Place the chocolate dipped balls on a baking sheet covered with a wax paper.

9. Refrigerate for about an hour or until set.

10. Serve chilled.

11. Enjoy!

Delicious Gluten Free Layer Bars

Serves: 15

Ingredients

- 3 ½ ounces sweetened flaked coconut, divided
- 3 ounces semisweet chocolate chips
- 1/2 cup butterscotch chips
- 1/4 pound unsalted peanuts
- 1/2 (14 ounce) can sweetened condensed milk
- 1/4 cup sliced almonds

Directions

1. Crank up your oven to 350 degrees Fahrenheit (about 175 degrees Celsius) and let it preheat for about 20 minutes. Grease a12 inches by 8 inches baking pan with some oil or spray t with some cooking spray.

2. Spread about 2/3rd of the flaked coconut in the bottom of the greased baking pan in an even layer.

3. Sprinkle a layer of butterscotch morsels over the flaked coconut layer, trying to keep the layer even.

4. Top the butterscotch morsels with a layer of chocolate chips.

5. Add in the peanuts in one last final layer over the chocolate chips.

6. Carefully pour the condensed milk over the layers, taking care that you do not disturb the layers that you have created.

7. Add the almonds on the top, followed by the leftover flaked coconut.

8. Pop the baking dish into the preheated oven and bake for about 20 to 30 minutes or until the coconut on the top looked toasted.

9. Remove the pan from the oven and cool completely before removing from the pan.

10. Cut into cubes and serve or store in an airtight jar.

11. Enjoy!

Delicious Chocolate and Cream Cheese Fudge

Serves: 32

Ingredients

- 3 ounces cream cheese, softened
- ¼ teaspoon vanilla extract
- 1/8 teaspoon salt
- 2 cups confectioners' sugar, sifted
- 2/3 cup and 1 tablespoon chopped walnuts
- 2 (1 ounce) squares unsweetened chocolate

Directions

1. Line a 5 inches by 5 inches baking dish with some heavy-duty aluminum foil.

2. Place the chocolate squares in a heat safe bowl and place it over a double boiler. Ensure that the bottom of the bowl does not touch the surface of the water.

3. Once the chocolate has melted, take it off the heat and cool it until it reaches room temperature.

4. Place the cream cheese in a medium sized bowl. Use an electric beater to beat it until the cream cheese has a smooth and lump free texture.

5. Add the confectioner's sugar in batches and beat vigorously between each addition so that all the sugar is well incorporated.

6. Pour the melted chocolate into the bowl and mix well.

7. Add in the walnuts and mix lightly.

8. Pour the prepared mix into the lined pan.

9. Refrigerate the fudge for 2 hours or until the fudge is firm to touch.

10. Cut the fudge into squares and serve or store in an airtight jar.

11. Enjoy!

Delicious Gluten Free Orange Cake

Serves: 8

Ingredients

- 1 whole orange with peel
- ½ pinch saffron powder (optional)
- 3 eggs
- 10 tablespoons white sugar
- 10 tablespoons finely ground almonds (almond meal)
- ¼ teaspoon baking powder
- ½ teaspoon finely chopped candied orange peel (optional)

Directions

1. Place the orange in a medium sized saucepan and pour water over the orange; enough to cover the orange. Heat the saucepan over a high flame until the water is bubbling.

2. Reduce the heat to a medium low and continue heating for about 1 and half to 2 hours. Check the orange every half an hour to ensure that there is enough cooking liquid in the pan and the cooking liquid doesn't completely dry out.

3. Cool the orange to room temperature. Cut open the orange and pick the seeds out of it. Process it in a food processor or blender until it resembles a coarse paste.

4. Crank up your oven to 375 degrees Fahrenheit (about 190 degrees Celsius) and let it preheat for about 20 minutes. Grease an 8-inch round cake pan with some butter or oil and line it with a parchment paper.

5. Place the eggs in a large mixing bowl and add the sugar to it. Using an electric beater beat the eggs for about 10 minutes or until they thicken up and become pale.

6. Add the baking powder and saffron (if using) to the eggs and mix well.

7. Pour the pureed orange into the egg mix and stir until incorporated.

8. Add the almond meal to the egg and orange puree mix in batches, mixing well after each addition. Add in the candied orange peel, if using, and mix well.

9. Pour the batter into the prepared baking tin.

10. Pop the cake into the preheated oven and bake for an hour or until a toothpick

inserted in the center of the cake comes out clean.

11. Remove the pan from the oven and cool the cake in the pan for about 10 minutes.

12. Run a warm knife around the edge of the pan to release it from the pan's edges.

13. Turn onto a serving plate.

14. Serve warm or completely cool.

15. Enjoy!

Gluten Free Coconut Macaroons

Serves: 30

Ingredients

- 1 ¼ cups shredded coconut
- 3 egg whites
- ½ cup white sugar
- 1 ½ teaspoons cornstarch
- ¾ cup halved red candied cherries
- 1/8 teaspoon almond extract

Directions

1. Crank up your oven to 350 degrees Fahrenheit (about 175 degrees Celsius) and let it preheat for about 20 minutes. Grease a cookie sheet with some butter or oil and line it with a parchment paper.
2. Combine the cornstarch and sugar together in a small mixing bowl. Whisk using a wire whisk until well combined.
3. Combine the egg whites with almond extract in a large metal bowl.
4. Add water to a deep pan and heat over a high flame until the water is simmering. Place the metal bowl with the egg whites on the pan with the simmering water.
5. Add the sugar and cornstarch mix to the egg whites and mix well.
6. Using an electric mixer whip the egg whites for about 15 to 20 minutes or until they become stiff and thick.
7. Add in the coconut and mix lightly so that the egg whites do not fall flat.
8. Take the bowl off heat and set aside to cool for a few minutes.
9. Transfer the mixture into a pastry bag that has been fitted with a large star tip.
10. Pipe out the cookies on the lined baking sheet at 1 to 1 ½ inch intervals and place ½ a cherry on each cookie.
11. Pop the baking sheet into the preheated oven and bake for about 20 to 22 minutes or until the cookies have a light golden brown exterior.
12. Let the cookies cool on the baking sheet for a few minutes before transferring them onto a wire rack to cool.
13. Serve warm or cool completely so that they become crispy.
14. Enjoy!

Gluten Free Flourless Chocolate Cake

Serves: 8

Ingredients

- 1/4 cup water
- 6 tablespoons white sugar
- 1/8 teaspoon salt
- 9 (1 ounce) squares bittersweet chocolate
- 3 eggs
- 1/2 cup unsalted butter

Directions

1. Crank up your oven to 300 degrees Fahrenheit (about 150 degrees Celsius) and let it preheat for about 20 minutes. Grease an 8-inch round cake pan with some butter or oil and line it with a parchment paper.
2. Combine the water, sugar and salt together in a small saucepan. Heat the pan over a medium high flame until the sugar is completely dissolved in the water. Keep aside.
3. Place the chocolate squares in a heat safe bowl and place it over a double boiler. Ensure that the bottom of the bowl does not touch the surface of the water. Or place the chocolate in a microwave safe bowl and heat the chocolate in the microwave for 20-second intervals, stirring well after each interval.
4. Pour the melted chocolate into the bowl of a stand mixer.
5. Cut the butter into large chunks and add them to the bowl with the chocolate one at a time, beating well after each addition so that the butter is well incorporated.
6. Add in the hot sugar, salt and water mixture and beat well until well combined.
7. Add in the eggs, one at a time, whisking well after each addition, to ensure that the egg is well incorporated.
8. Pour this batter into the greased and lined pan and tap it lightly on the kitchen counter to rid it of the air bubbles.
9. Place the cake batter filled pan in a larger pan and pour in some boiling water into the larger pan until the water level touches the halfway mark of the cake filled pan.
10. Pop the cake with its water bath into the preheated oven and bake for about 45 to 50 minutes. The center will be slightly moist and wet.
11. Leave the cake to cool in the pan and transfer it to the refrigerator to chill for a few hours or overnight.
12. Dip the bottom of the cake tin in some hot water for about 10 to 15 seconds and invert the cake onto a serving plate.
13. Serve topped with some berries.
14. Enjoy!

Delicious Chocolate Meringue Cookies

Serves: 9

Ingredients

- 1 ½ egg whites
- ¼ teaspoon vanilla extract
- 1/8 teaspoon cream of tartar
- 1/3 cup white sugar
- 8 teaspoons semisweet chocolate chips
- 1 ½ teaspoons unsweetened cocoa powder

Directions

1. Crank up your oven to 300 degrees Fahrenheit (about 150 degrees Celsius) and let it preheat for about 20 minutes. Grease a cookie sheet with some butter or oil and line it with a parchment paper.

2. Combine the egg whites, vanilla extract and cream of tartar together in a large mixing bowl. Beat with a hand blender until the egg whites form soft peaks.

3. Gradually add the sugar to the egg white mix and whisk until the whites form peaks and the mixture becomes glossy.

4. Mix the chocolate chips and cocoa to the mix and gently fold until incorporated.

5. Scoop about a tablespoon of the batter onto the prepared cookie sheet.

6. Pop the cookie sheet into the preheated oven and bake for about 30 to 35 minutes or until the cookies start drying out around the edges.

7. Cool the cookies on the baking sheet for a few minutes before transferring them onto a wire rack for further cooling.

8. Serve them immediately or store them an airtight jar for consumption later.

9. Enjoy!

Zingy Lemon Soufflé

Serves: 2

Ingredients

- 1/2 egg
- 2 tablespoons superfine sugar or castor sugar
- 1/2 large lemon, zested and juiced
- 1/2 teaspoon cornstarch
- 1 ½ egg whites
- 1 tablespoon unsalted butter, cut into cubes
- 7 ½ teaspoons superfine sugar or castor sugar
- 1/2 large lemon, zested and juiced
- 1 ½ egg yolks
- 1 tablespoon confectioners' sugar for dusting

Directions

1. Crank up your oven to 350 degrees Fahrenheit (about 175 degrees Celsius) and let it preheat for about 20 minutes.

2. Pour the egg into a medium sized saucepan and whisk well. Add in the zest and juice from half the lemon, 2 tablespoons sugar and cornstarch and mix until well combined.

3. Heat the saucepan over a medium low flame and constantly stir while the mixture cooks and slowly thickens.

4. Reduce the flame to low and whisk the mixture for another minute or so.

5. Take the pan off the heat and add the butter to the saucepan and mix until the butter is incorporated.

6. Spoon the mixture into 2 large or 4 small ramekins. Keep aside.

7. Pour the egg whites into a large metal or glass bowl and whisk them using an electric mixer. Once the egg whites are whipped enough to hold soft peaks, add in about 3 teaspoons of the sugar and continue whisking until the egg whites become stiff.

8. Add the remaining 4-½ teaspoons of sugar to the egg yolks. Add in the remaining lemon zest and lemon juice and whisk the egg yolks.

9. Add a few tablespoons of the egg whites to the egg yolks to make them a lighter.

Then add all the egg whites to the egg yolk mix and fold gently until incorporated. Do not over mix or the egg whites will lose their fluffiness.

10. Spoon the prepared mix into the ramekins and gently run a finger around the inside of each ramekin rim.

11. Arrange the ramekins on a baking sheet and place the baking sheet in the preheated oven. Bake for about 17 to 20 minutes or until the tops of the soufflés puff out and become golden brown.

12. Cool the soufflés for a few minutes before serving.

13. Enjoy!

Gluten Free Peanut Butter Cookies

Serves: 30

Ingredients

- 1 ½ cups chopped pecans (optional)
- 2 cups peanut butter
- 4 eggs, beaten
- 2 cups white sugar
- 2 cups semi-sweet chocolate chips (optional)

Directions

1. Crank up your oven to 350 degrees Fahrenheit (about 175 degrees Celsius) and let it preheat for about 20 minutes. Grease a cookie sheet with some butter or oil and line it with a parchment paper.

2. Add the peanut butter, sugar and eggs together to a large mixing bowl and mix well until smooth.

3. Add in the chocolate chips and pecans to the mix if using.

4. Scoop about a tablespoon of the dough and place it on the prepared baking sheet.

5. Repeat with the remaining batter, leaving about 1 to 1 ½ inch of space between two cookies.

6. Pop the cookie sheet into the oven and bake for about 12 to 15 minutes or until the edges of the cookies start drying out.

7. Cool the cookies on the cookie sheet for a few minutes before transferring them onto a wire rack for cooling.

8. Serve immediately or store in an airtight container to eat later.

9. Enjoy!

Gooey Black Bean Brownies

Serves: 8

Ingredients

- 1/2 (15.5 ounce) can black beans, rinsed and drained
- 4 ½ teaspoons vegetable oil
- 1 ½ eggs
- 2 tablespoons cocoa powder
- 1/2 teaspoon vanilla extract
- 1/2 pinch salt
- 10 tablespoons white sugar
- 1/4 cup milk chocolate chips (optional)
- 1/2 teaspoon instant coffee (optional)

Directions

1. Crank up your oven to 350 degrees Fahrenheit (about 175 degrees Celsius) and let it preheat for about 20 minutes. Grease an 8 inches by 8 inches baking tin with some butter or oil and line it with a parchment paper.

2. Place the black beans and eggs together in the jar of a blender. Blitz until well combined.

3. Add in the oil, salt, sugar, cocoa powder, vanilla extract and instant coffee (if using). Continue blending to form a smooth batter.

4. Pour the prepared batter into the prepared baking tin and sprinkle the chocolate chips over the batter (if using).

5. Pop the baking dish into the preheated oven and bake the brownies for about 30 to 35 minutes or until the top of the brownie dries out and edges of the brownie start pulling away from the sides of the baking pan.

6. Cool the brownie in the pan for about 10 to 12 minutes before turning the brownie onto a wire rack.

7. Cool and serve with some gluten free chocolate sauce or gluten free vanilla ice cream.

8. Enjoy!

Gluten Free Garbanzo Bean Chocolate Cake

Serves: 6

Ingredients

- 3/4 cup semisweet chocolate chips
- 2 eggs
- 1/2 (19 ounce) can garbanzo beans, rinsed and drained
- 6 tablespoons white sugar
- 1 ½ teaspoons confectioners' sugar for dusting
- 1/4 teaspoon baking powder

Directions

1. Crank up your oven to 350 degrees Fahrenheit (about 175 degrees Celsius) and let it preheat for about 20 minutes. Grease an 8-inch round cake pan with some butter or oil and line it with a parchment paper.

2. Place the chocolate squares in a heat safe bowl and place it over a double boiler. Ensure that the bottom of the bowl does not touch the surface of the water. Or place the chocolate in a microwave safe bowl and heat the chocolate in the microwave for 20-second intervals, stirring well after each interval.

3. Place the eggs and beans together in the jar of a blender or food processor. Blitz until you get a smooth paste.

4. Add the baking powder and sugar to the bean and egg mixture and continue blending until mixed.

5. Add the melted chocolate to the blender and continue blending until all the chocolate is well incorporated.

6. Pour the batter into the prepared baking tin.

7. Pop the baking tin into the preheated oven and bake for about 35 to 45 minutes.

8. Cool the cake in the pan for about 15 to 20 minutes.

9. Remove the cake from the tin and cool on a wire rack before transferring the cake on to a serving plate.

10. Dust the cake with some confectioner's sugar and serve immediately.

11. Enjoy!

Creamy Gluten Free Rice Pudding

Serves: 6

Ingredients

- 4 cups milk
- 1/2 cup uncooked long-grain white rice
- 1/2 cup white sugar
- 1 ½ eggs, lightly beaten
- 1/8 teaspoon salt
- Ground cinnamon, to taste
- 2 tablespoons milk
- 1 teaspoon vanilla extract

Directions

1. Combine the 4 cups milk, rice and sugar together in a large saucepan. Heat the saucepan over a medium low flame.

2. Cover the saucepan with a lid and let the milk simmer for an hour or so. Make sure you give the milk a stir every 15 minutes. Take the saucepan off heat and set it aside for about 10 to 15 minutes.

3. In a small mixing bowl, add in the eggs, salt, 2 tablespoons milk and vanilla extract together. Whisk well until well combined.

4. Pour the mix into the rice and milk mixture and mix well.

5. Place the saucepan over a low flame and mix constantly, while cooking it for about 2 to 3 minutes.

6. Pour the pudding into an 8-inches by 12-inches baking dish and cover the dish with some plastic wrap. Fold the plastic wrap back around the corners so that the steam from the baking dish can escape.

7. When the pudding is significantly cooler and close to room temperature, remove the plastic wrap.

8. Sprinkle the cinnamon over the pudding.

9. Cover the baking dish with a fresh plastic wrap and make sure it is tightly covered.

10. Refrigerate for a few hours, or even overnight, before serving.

11. Spoon into individual bowls and serve chilled.

12. Enjoy!

Cream Cheese Mints

Serves: 8

Ingredients

- Any color food coloring paste (optional)
- 1/2 (3 ounce) package cream cheese, softened
- 1 ½ cups confectioners' sugar
- 1 ½ teaspoons butter, softened
- 1 drop peppermint oil

Directions

1. Combine the cream cheese, confectioner's sugar and butter together in a large mixing bowl.

2. Add the peppermint oil to the mix and whisk using an electric beater until the batter is smooth and lump free.

3. If you wish to add some color to your mints, add some food color to the batter or leave it white.

4. Lightly oil your palms and fingers and scoop about a teaspoon of the batter in your hands.

5. Roll the batter into a small ball and place it on a baking sheet covered with waxed paper. Repeat with the remaining batter.

6. Lightly flatten the balls using a fork that has been dipped in some confectioner's sugar.

7. Let the mints dry out for about 2 to 3 hours and then transfer the mints to the refrigerator or freezer.

8. Serve chilled.

9. Enjoy!

Chapter 10: Common Units of Conversion in the Kitchen

While the whole world uses metric conversions that use weight as a measuring unit, Americans measure everything by their volume. This often causes a little confusion, especially in the kitchen. This chapter contains some common unit conversions as well as other conversions (such as temperature conversions) that are often needed in the kitchen.

US Dry Volume Measurements

Equivalent	Measure
Dash	1/16 tsp
Pinch	1/8 tsp
1 tbsp.	3 tsp
2 tbsp.	1/8 cup
4 tbsp.	1/4 cup
5 tbsp.	1/3 cup
8 tbsp.	1/2 cup
12 tbsp.	3/4 cup
16 tbsp.	1 cup
16 oz.	1 lb.

US liquid volume measurements

Equivalent	Measure
1 cup	8 fl. oz.
2 cups	1 pint
2 pints	1 quart
1 gallon	4 quarts

US to Metric Conversions

Equivalent	Measure
5 ml	1 tsp
15 ml	1 tbsp.
30 ml	1 fl. oz.
50 ml	1/5 cup
240 ml	1 cup
470 ml	2 cups
.95 liters	4 cups
3.8 liters	4 quarts
28 g	1 oz.
100 g	3.5 oz.
454 g	1 lb.
1 kg	2.20 lb.

Metric to US Conversions
Oven Temperature Conversions

Celsius	Fahrenheit	Gas Mark
140° C	275° F	1 cool
150° C	300° F	2
165° C	325° F	3 very moderate
180° C	350° F	4 moderate
190° C	375° F	5
200° C	400° F	6 moderately hot
220° C	425° F	7 hot
230° C	450° F	9
240° C	475° F	10 very hot

Conclusion

Going gluten free can be extremely healthy for you in the long run. It can also help you lose extra pounds when followed with some moderation. But, as re-iterated in this book repeatedly, going gluten free doesn't mean that you can eat anything and everything and not pay attention to their calorie content or their portions. Just because you cut the glutinous foods from your diet, it doesn't mean that you are going to magically start dropping those extra pounds!

Rather, having the mindset the every and any gluten free food is diet food, influences your mind and you end up eating more than your require. It is extremely important that you keep track of what you eat and be aware of your eating habits.

The best way to keep an eye on what you eat and keep an adequate track is to note down everything that you eat – either in a food journal or in a food tracker app. It is important to keep a track of the *ingredients*, the portion and the time at which you ate that particular food.

At the end of each week go through everything that you ate – you will be able to adequately judge which foods you are eating too much of and which foods you are not eating enough of. You will also be able to pinpoint the exact time when you start falling off the wagon!

From this book you can see how the gluten free diet is good for your health and that you can not only drop those pesky extra pounds by following it, but also relieve a lot of your body issues, such as insomnia, digestive issues, skin issues, etc.

With rising popularity and growing demands, there are many gluten free versions of unhealthy foods available in the market. It is very important to keep in mind that the gluten free diet is no magic diet and not everything labeled to be "gluten free" is good for your health. Make it a habit to read labels carefully and even get in touch with manufacturers if you are not sure of certain products. Even if foods are gluten free, it doesn't make them any less unhealthy!

So, even while following the gluten free diet, it is important to avoid all the highly processed and unhealthy foods. Stick to the "real" and healthy foods, such as fruits, vegetables, dairy, meats, nuts, seeds, beans, etc. and you will reap the benefits in no time at all.

I would like to thank you once again for purchasing this book and I hope you found the content of this book useful!

Made in the USA
Middletown, DE
18 February 2018